PEDIATRIC

DEVELOPMENTAL

DIAGNOSIS

Editors

William K. Frankenburg, M.D.
Director, John F. Kennedy Child Development Center
Professor, Pediatrics and Preventive Medicine
School of Medicine
University of Colorado Health Sciences Center

Susan M. Thornton, M.S.
Consulting Writer and Editor
Coordinator, Physicians Training Program
John F. Kennedy Child Development Center
School of Medicine
University of Colorado Health Sciences Center

Marlin E. Cohrs
Media Director
John F. Kennedy Child Development Center
School of Medicine
University of Colorado Health Sciences Center

1981
Thieme-Stratton, Inc., New York
Georg Thieme Verlag Stuttgart • New York

Publisher: Thieme-Stratton Inc.
381 Park Avenue South
New York, New York 10016

PEDIATRIC DEVELOPMENTAL DIAGNOSIS

ISBN 0-86577-019-0

Last digit is print number 9 8 7 6 5 4 3

DEDICATION

This book is dedicated to the millions of developmentally disadvantaged children in the United States and the world. It is hoped that this book will make physicians increasingly aware of some of the common causes of developmental problems in childhood, and thereby will encourage physicians to promote the health and development of all children. It is these same physicians, given appropriate orientation, who can enhance the quality of life of handicapped children and their families, and who can help these children realize their potential to become major contributors to the societies in which they live.

PREFACE

This book has evolved over the past five years; it came into being because of the need we saw for a basic text to train primary care physicians to perform diagnostic evaluations of children suspected of having developmental problems. Although most pediatric training programs include elements of such a diagnostic evaluation, few attempt to provide the resident or busy practitioner with a complete protocol to follow when such a suspect child is encountered.

The result is that many physicians, not knowing how to evaluate such children, refer them to a diagnostic center without attempting to evaluate the children themselves; alternatively, they refer children to a specialist such as a speech pathologist or occupational therapist depending upon the most prominent presenting complaint. The former approach of unnecessarily referring suspect children is not only costly to the child's parents and/or society, but also results in long waiting lists at diagnostic centers. The second approach—referral to specialists for assessment of the major presenting complaint—may preclude the discovery of other problems which may be more significant. These approaches are in sharp contrast to the protocols that primary care physicians follow in evaluating and treating far more rare presenting symptoms such as seizures, growth retardation, and fever disorders.

In the past few years, with the recognition of the value of early intervention and treatment of children with developmental problems, the recommendation of developmental screening by professional organizations and legislation has become almost universal. As a consequence, an ever-growing number of infants and preschool-age children are presumptively identified through screening and are referred to their physician for an evaluation. This book's goal is to teach the primary care physician—whether a pediatrician or family physician—to perform a basic diagnostic evaluation. Such comprehensive evaluations are essential, for without a diagnosis developed through ruling out all the major contributing factors, a complete and appropriate habilitation program cannot be designed.

This book presents the primary care practitioner and resident with a rationale for early diagnosis and habilitation; a practical approach to the comprehensive evaluation of children with developmental problems (including indications for referral to other specialists); suggested ways of sharing evaluation results with parents of the handicapped child; and methods by which the professional can work with schools and community agencies to ensure the optimal education and treatment for the child.

Since the need for such training is almost universal, the authors have attempted to develop a brief protocol for conducting diagnostic evaluations. Such a protocol has not previously been attempted and there is no uniformity of opinion as to what procedures and criteria should be used to evaluate young children suspected of having developmental delays. The final protocol or algorithm that evolved is but one approach; without doubt most physicians having experience in developmental diagnosis might prefer a somewhat different approach. It is, therefore, important for the reader to realize that the protocol is designed as a "start" for the busy generalist who is faced with a child who is suspected of a developmental delay. The "start" should suffice for the evaluation of suspect children who have relatively simple developmental problems. For the remaining children—perhaps 20 percent of the handicapped population presenting with more complex problems—this evaluation process will serve as a base which must be supplemented by more extensive consultations. Generally, the more complex the problem, the more it will be necessary for the primary care physician to involve specialists with more extensive training in this field.

It would be presumptuous to edit such a book without recognizing its limitations. First, the text is not intended for physicians who are already knowledgeable in developmental diagnosis. Second, this book is intended to impart information; it cannot teach the skills that are so essential to the physician but that only come through practice. The limitations of the evaluation protocol have been discussed; we fully recognize that the protocol may change as better evaluation techniques are identified.

The reader should be aware that this text represents but one part of a tutored videotape training program. The tutors* (located across the United States and in several other countries) are physicians already experienced in pediatric developmental diagnosis. They have undergone special orientation sessions to acquaint them with methods of utilizing the training program to make it most effective. The tutors present videotapes that contain brief lectures, demonstration of techniques, and case demonstrations; in addition, the tutors lead discussions, answer questions, supervise practicums, and discuss local resources. This text is used in the videotaped training program and is designed to remind participating physicians of the process of diagnostic evaluation. The total training time for the course is 26 hours; 20 hours of videotaped presentation is followed by a practicum period during which the participants practice their newly acquired skills before meeting again for a six-hour period of review with the tutor. Evaluation data from the first 220 physicians undergoing this training program were very favorable in that each of the 17 lessons was rated between good and very good, and more than 90 percent of physicians taking the course stated that they would recommend it to other physicians.

This text is a result of contributions of many people who have either written lessons or critiqued them; many of these persons are listed on the acknowledgment page. We wish to express our special thanks for the comprehensive critiques by Drs. Clifford J. Sells, Forrest C. Bennett, Christopher Williams, and Paul Pearson, each of whom have many years of experience in teaching developmental diagnosis and who spent three days reviewing the content of the training program. In addition, many helpful comments and suggestions by the tutors (93 as of this writing) were also incorporated into the text. Last but not least, the candid comments by the more than 700 busy

---

*To obtain the name of the tutor residing nearest to you, contact one of the editors at the JFK Child Development Center by calling 303-394-8251.

practitioners who took the course during its first year of dissemination have been most helpful in assuring that the protocol was appropriate for its intended audience.

The preparation of this text (and the training program as a whole) has been an immensely challenging effort, and one which has provided much personal growth and satisfaction to us. It is our hope that this book will prove useful to primary care physicians, and that it may contribute in a small measure to improving the quality of life for handicapped children and their families.

William K. Frankenburg, M.D.
Susan M. Thornton, M.S.
Marlin E. Cohrs

CONTENTS

CONTRIBUTORS

FORREST C. BENNETT, M.D.
Assistant Professor of Pediatrics and Director of Medical Education, Clinical Training Unit/CDMRC, University of Washington Health Science Center

RATIONALE FOR EARLY IDENTIFICATION AND TREATMENT

LAWRENCE H. BERNSTEIN, M.D.
Clinical Assistant Professor of Pediatrics and Neurology, University of Colorado Health Sciences Center

NEUROLOGICAL EVALUATION

FLORENCE BERMAN BLAGER, Ph.D.
Associate Professor of Otolaryngology and Psychiatry, University of Colorado Health Sciences Center, and Chief of Speech Pathology and Audiology, John F. Kennedy Child Development Center

SPEECH AND LANGUAGE EVALUATION

ROGER V. CADOL, M.D.
Colonel, Medical Corps, U.S. Army, and Chief of Child Development Section, Fitzsimons Army Medical Center

MEDICAL HISTORY AND PHYSICAL EXAMINATION

DONALD E. COOK, M.D.
Pediatrician in private practice, and Chairman of the American Academy of Pediatrics' School Health Committee

COMMUNITY RESOURCES

ALMA W. FANDAL
Developmental Screening Coordinator, John F. Kennedy Child Development Center, University of Colorado Health Sciences Center

DEVELOPMENTAL SCREENING

PETER S. FANNING, Ed.D.
  Executive Director of Special Education Services, Colorado Department of Education,
  Denver, Colorado

  EDUCATIONAL PLANNING

HENRY L. FISCHER, Ph.D.
  Private clinical psychologist with a specialty in working with developmentally handicapped
  children

  ENVIRONMENTAL EVALUATION (SUPPLEMENTAL READING)

WILLIAM K. FRANKENBURG, M.D.
  Director, John F. Kennedy Child Development Center and Professor of Pediatrics and
  Preventive Medicine, University of Colorado Health Sciences Center

  INTRODUCTION TO DIAGNOSTIC EVALUATION
  DEVELOPMENTAL SCREENING
  PRACTICUM

MELINDA B. KEMPER, M.A.
  Coordinator, Newborn Followup Program, Department of Perinatology, Children's Hospital,
  Denver, Colorado

  DEVELOPMENTAL SCREENING

HAROLD P. MARTIN, M.D.
  Associate Professor of Pediatrics and Psychiatry, University of Colorado Health Sciences
  Center

  ABUSE AND NEGLECT EVALUATION
  PARENT CONFERENCES

EDWARD R. McCABE, M.D.
  Assistant Professor of Pediatrics and Biochemistry, Biophysics and Genetics, University of
  Colorado Health Sciences Center

  METABOLIC EVALUATION

JOHN MELCHER
  Supervisor of Early Childhood Programs for Handicapped Children and Director of the State
  Implementation Grant for Early Childhood (Handicapped), Department of Public Instruction,
  Madison, Wisconsin

  EDUCATIONAL PLANNING

JERRY NORTHERN, Ph.D.
Professor of Otolaryngology and Head, Audiology Division, University of Colorado Health Sciences Center

AUDIOLOGICAL EVALUATION

DONOUGH O'BRIEN, M.D., F.R.C.P.
Professor of Pediatrics, University of Colorado Health Sciences Center

METABOLIC EVALUATION

STEVEN POOLE, M.D.
Assistant Professor of Family Medicine and Pediatrics, University of Colorado Health Sciences Center

INTEGRATION OF DIAGNOSTIC FINDINGS

JAMES SPRAGUE, M.D.
Assistant Professor of Ophthalmology, University of Colorado Health Sciences Center

OPHTHALMOLOGICAL EVALUATION

EVA SUJANSKY, M.D.
Director, Genetics Unit, and Associate Professor of Pediatrics and Biochemistry, Biophysics and Genetics, University of Colorado Health Sciences Center

GENETIC EVALUATION

GORDON ULREY, Ph.D.
Assistant Professor of Clinical Psychology, John F. Kennedy Child Development Center, University of Colorado Health Sciences Center

PSYCHOLOGICAL EVALUATION

ACKNOWLEDGMENTS

This training program has been under development for more than four years, and has involved persons listed below as well as others too numerous to mention. Noted specialists from many fields have given generously of their time and expertise to bring this project to fruition.

The editors wish to express their deep appreciation for the efforts and enthusiasm of all those who helped make this project possible. In particular we wish to thank: Carolyn L. Mears for editing early versions of this text and the final bibliographies; Jay S. Lawson for artwork; and Patti A. Thedens for typing.

Rationale for Early Intervention
    Nicholas J. Anastasiow, Ph.D.
    Graham M. Sterritt, Ph.D.
    Brian McNulty

Medical History and Physical Examination
    Roger M. Barkin, M.D.

Ophthalmological Evaluation
    Robert A. Sargent, M.D.
    Malcolm A. Tarkanian, M.D.
    John S. Barker, M.D.
    Max Kaplan, M.D.

Audiological Evaluation
    Janet M. Zarnoch, M.A.
    Larry Webster, Ph.D.

Speech and Language Evaluation
    R. L. Schiefelbusch, Ph.D.
    Calvin Knobeloch, Ph.D.
    Thelma D. Turner, M.A.

Neurological and Neuromotor Evaluation
    Mary Anne Guggenheim, M.D.
    Janet E. Young, M.D., R.P.T.
    Patricia Kurtz, R.P.T.
    Roger C. Hindle, M.D.
    Peggy C. Ferry, M.D.
    David A. Stumpf, M.D.
    Robert E. Eiben, M.D.
    Diane Meckstroth, R.P.T.
    Brian Grabert, M.D.
    Lillian Pardo, M.D.

Metabolic Evaluation
    Selma E. Snyderman, M.D.
    George N. Donnell, M.D.
    Louis J. Elsas, II, M.D.
    Parvin Justice, Ph.D.

Genetic Evaluation
    Lewis B. Holmes, M.D.
    Arthur Robinson, M.D.
    Kurt Hirschhorn, M.D.
    Herbert A. Lubs, M.D.
    Vincent Ricardi, M.D.
    Ann C. M. Smith, M.A.

Psychological Evaluation
    Henry Coppolillo, M.D.
    Josiah B. Dodds, Ph.D.
    Henry L. Fischer, Ph.D.
    William van Doorninck, Ph.D.
    James Q. Simmons, III, M.D.
    Irving Philips, M.D.
    Norman R. Bernstein, M.D.
    Nancy M. Robinson, Ph.D.
    Carolyn S. Schroeder, Ph.D.
    Ann M. Garner, Ph.D.
    Sally J. Rogers, Ph.D.

Abuse and Neglect Evaluation
    Susan L. Scheurer, M.D.
    Robin L. Hansen, M.D.

Parent Conferences
    Deborah K. Bublitz, M.D.
    Melvin H. Weiner, M.D.
    Lee S. Thompson, M.D.
    Herbert Josepher, M.D.
    Lawrence I. Waldman, M.D.

Educational Planning
    Edward Sontag, Ph.D.
    Elizabeth D. Gunzelman
    Herbert Goldstein, Ed.D.
    Mary Curtis, M.A.

Community Resources
    Daniel J. Gossert, A.C.S.W.
    Pamela Landon, M.S.W.
    Alice Kitt

Others
    Doris Haar
    Dave Hibbard, M.D.
    Nancy Hester, M.N.
    Forrest C. Bennett, M.D.

Paul H. Pearson, M.D.
Clifford J. Sells, M.D.
Christopher Williams, M.D.
David Irby, Ph.D.
Jolene Constance

PART I

Chapter 1

Goal To present the objectives of the training program, and to describe the manner in which it is organized.

Objectives At the end of this chapter, the physician should be able to:
- state the objectives of the training program;
- describe the role of the tutor in the training program, and the two roles which the program will prepare the physician to fill.

IDENTIFICATION OF CHILDREN SUSPECTED OF DEVELOPMENTAL DELAYS

INTRODUCTION TO DIAGNOSTIC EVALUATION

By
WILLIAM K. FRANKENBURG, M.D.

I. Introduction
   A. It will be necessary to vastly expand this country's diagnostic capacity if mandated screening and treatment objectives are to be met.
   B. Primary care physicians who complete this training program will be in a position to evaluate 80 percent of those children who are suspect on screening.
II. The Physician's Role
   A. The first role the physician may chose to play is the traditional one of case manager; the second role is that of a consultant serving as a member of a diagnostic team.
   B. This training program has been designed to prepare the physician to serve either role.
III. Objectives of the Training Program
   The objectives of the program are:
   1. To teach physicians to identify problems which require medical treatment and those which have implications for genetic counseling;
   2. To assist physicians in identifying emotional and psychological disorders that are secondary to deprivation;
   3. To teach physicians when to refer a child to consultants;
   4. To assist physicians in identifying concurrent health problems which may deter remediation efforts if left untreated;
   5. To teach physicians how to assemble diverse findings;
   6. To impart to physicians effective techniques for sharing findings with parents;
   7. To suggest ways physicians can optimize a handicapped child's development through knowledge of the schools and community resources.
IV. The Tutor's Role
   A. This training program requires participation of a tutor, who will promote discussions, offer practice activities to the students, and so forth.
   B. It is requested that students complete evaluation forms at the end of each lesson to assist in assembling the most effective training program.
V. Summary

INTRODUCTION

During the past few years there has been nation-wide acceptance of the importance of early identification and treatment of children with developmental disabilities. As a result, universal and periodic developmental screening has been recommended by professional associations, and legislated by federal and state governments. If the mandated screening and treatment objectives are to be met, it will be necessary to vastly expand this country's diagnostic capacity so that each handicapped child receives the appropriate therapy and education.

This training program attempts to remedy some of the problems related to the national scarcity of diagnostic services. Primary care physicians who complete the following training program will be in a position to evaluate 80 percent of those children who are suspect on screening. The remaining 20 percent of those children who have complex problems might then be referred to regional developmental evaluation clinics, such as university affiliated centers and others which specialize in serving handicapped children. This program is designed for the busy generalist physician, whether a family physician or pediatrician; it recognizes the diverse interests of these practitioners, the pressure to see many patients, and the economics of practice.

THE PHYSICIAN'S ROLE

It is anticipated that primary care physicians will play one of two roles in the diagnostic process. The first is the traditional one of case manager, a role that physicians have served in the past when confronted with a perplexing diagnostic case or a multiply-handicapped child. In this role, the physician would perform a primary diagnostic evaluation, decide which examinations were needed, refer the child to consultants, and interpret test results to the parents.

A second role the physician may play is that of a consultant serving as a member of a diagnostic team. In this situation, case management may be under the direction of a local community agency (such as a school).

Local circumstances and the physician's own inclination will generally determine which of these roles he or she will play. This training program has been designed to prepare the physician to serve either as a case manager or as a member of the diagnostic team.

OBJECTIVES OF THE TRAINING PROGRAM

In addition, this program is intended to teach both medical residents and practitioners basic information required to evaluate children who are suspect on developmental screening. The specific objectives of the program are:

1. to teach physicians to identify problems that require specific medical treatment and those which have implications for genetic counseling, so as to minimize the recurrence of such handicaps;
2. to assist physicians in identifying emotional and psychological disorders that are secondary to deprivation, since they require prompt and specific therapy;
3. to teach physicians when to refer a child to consultants such as psychologists, speech pathologists, physical and occupational therapists, and so on;
4. to assist physicians in identifying concurrent health problems, which though not responsible for the child's developmental delay, may nevertheless deter remediation efforts if left untreated;
5. to teach physicians how to assemble the diverse findings of the case history, of the medical examination, and of the consultants so that a comprehensive individualized therapeutic plan can be developed;
6. to impart to physicians effective techniques for sharing findings with parents;
7. to suggest ways in which physicians can optimize a handicapped child's development through knowledge of the schools and community resources.

To meet these objectives, this training program has been divided into two parts. The first pertains to the rationale for early identification and developmental screening. The second part deals with the diagnostic process, the collation of data, the presentation of data to parents, and the physician's involvement in educational planning and the use of community resources.

THE TUTOR'S ROLE

This training program is not intended to be self-instructional; rather it requires the participation of a tutor, who will interrupt the videotaped presentations to answer questions, promote discussions, and offer practice activities to the students. An additional role of the tutor is to discuss the use of local resources.

SUMMARY

The physician who completes this training program should realize that actual skill in developmental diagnosis comes only with practice. It is like learning to ski; one cannot master the slopes by watching a film or reading a book. To be sure, the fundamentals presented in a film or a book must be understood first, but the mastery of any skill is accomplished only with practice. In addition, to be most effective, such practice should be accompanied by periodic critiques by specialists.

Chapter 2

Goal
To develop an awareness that the effects of a developmental handicap on a child and the family can be reversed or ameliorated, especially if the handicap is identified at an early age.

Objectives
At the end of this chapter, the physician should be able to:
- cite specific examples of different types of early intervention and their relative merits;
- differentiate the two major subdivisions of mental retardation;
- discuss rational bases for early developmental intervention and how these may positively influence physicians' attitudes and practice patterns.

RATIONALE FOR EARLY
IDENTIFICATION AND TREATMENT

By

FORREST C. BENNETT, M.D.

I. Introduction
   A. The effectiveness of early intervention for actual or potential developmental disorders is the cornerstone on which developmental diagnosis and early identification efforts rest.
   B. Unfortunately, health care professionals all too frequently believe that nothing can be done for major disabilities or believe that mild delays will be outgrown.
   C. These attitudes can delay treatment of children with handicaps, and in some cases can seriously interfere with the eventual effectiveness of remediation efforts.
II. Generally Accepted Types of Early Intervention
   A. Newborn screening programs prevent mental retardation in cases of phenylketonuria and congenital hypothyroidism.
   B. Blind and/or deaf children require early stimulation and education to prevent functional mental retardation.
   C. Early physical therapy benefits infants and young children with cerebral palsy.
III. Two Major Types of Mental Retardation
   A. Mental retardation is not a single disease syndrome or symptom; it is rather a state of impairment which is recognized in the behavior of the individual.
   B. Severely impaired children, who frequently manifest overt brain damage, constitute about 11 percent of those children classified as retarded.
   C. Mildly impaired children, whose retardation often has a cultural-familial basis, constitute about 89 percent of children classified as retarded; this group might especially benefit from early developmental stimulation.
IV. Two Opposing Theories of Intellectual Development
   A. Jensen, stressing genetic and hereditary factors in the development of intellect, views environmental experiences as only a threshold variable.
   B. Bloom believes that the quality of the environment has a linear relationship to the development of intelligence.
   C. As a corollary, Bloom finds that about 50 percent of IQ differences at maturity can be explained by IQ differences at age four; thus environmental intervention has the greatest impact if begun during the early preschool years.
V. Intervention Programs Less Well-Accepted by Physicians
   A. Programs such as Project Head Start, designed for children at risk of developing cultural-familial retardation, are showing long-range benefits in academic achievement and reduction of school failure.
   B. Programs for developmentally disabled children, such as those

with Down Syndrome, are finding gains in language, learning skills, personal-social behavior, and overall family functioning.

VI. Bases for Early Intervention
  A. Early experiences influence all areas of development.
  B. Environmental experiences modify the developmental sequelae of perinatal distress.
  C. There may be critical periods during early life for the development of certain skills.
  D. Lack of early stimulation can lead to atrophy of sensory abilities and to developmental regression.
  E. Failure to remediate a handicap can produce secondary deficits in other areas of development.
  F. When recognition of a handicap is delayed, the cognitive gap between a delayed child and other children widens over time.
  G. Early intervention should be evaluated on the basis of reducing the effects of a handicapping condition, not on dramatically curing the condition.
  H. Parents need support and specific instructions for raising a handicapped child.

VII. Summary

INTRODUCTION

The effectiveness of early intervention for actual or potential developmental disorders is the cornerstone on which developmental diagnosis and early identification efforts rest. Child health professionals must become convinced there is something beneficial to offer developmentally delayed children and their families before they will conscientiously participate in routine developmental screening of all the infants and children in their care. Unfortunately, this important cornerstone frequently turns out to be instead the major stumbling block impeding wide-spread enthusiasm for and implementation of early developmental diagnosis.

Why should this be? Health care professionals all too frequently believe that early identification through screening, followed by diagnostic workups, is useless because early therapeutic and educational intervention for most developmental disabilities is useless. These professionals hold one of two basic attitudes. The first is a relatively hopeless and fatalistic attitude toward major disabilities, such as significant mental retardation. The second is a sentiment for allowing nature to take its course and giving the child with milder developmental delays, such as an early language deficit, the chance to outgrow the problem. Both attitudes can delay treatment of young children, and in some cases can seriously interfere with the eventual effectiveness of overall remediation programs. This chapter will attempt to respond to these pessimistic and skeptical attitudes toward early intervention efforts through a brief examination of different types of intervention strategies which formulate rational bases for early intervention.

GENERALLY ACCEPTED TYPES OF EARLY INTERVENTION

Newborn screening programs are currently mandated in most states for the very early detection of phenylketonuria, a genetic inborn error of amino acid metabolism with an incidence of about one in 12,000 live births. This condition brought new respect and interest to the field of mental retardation when it was discovered in the late 1950s and early 1960s that early dietary intervention, if begun as soon after birth as possible, could actually prevent the brain damage associated with this disorder. Thus, phenylketonuria was widely recognized as the first preventable cause of mental deficiency, and most physicians are interested in its early identification because of the proven effectiveness of early intervention.

Congenital hypothyroidism, an even more common cause of mental and physical retardation (one in 5,000 live births), has recently also been found to be potentially detectable by routine newborn blood screening. Here again the effectiveness of early intervention (via hormone replacement) to prevent subsequent mental deficiency is currently being documented.

Early intervention for young children with major sensory deficits, i.e., blind and/or deaf children, is also generally accepted by most physicians, even though identification of these special disabilities is often delayed. A blind and deaf child untreated until the age of six will probably spend life in a dependent state of functional mental retardation. It has been found that when congenitally blind children are not provided with stimulation to compensate for the lack of sight, they frequently develop stereotypical hand behaviors, rocking, swaying, mutism, or echolalic speech and are often suspected of having brain damage and/or infantile autism. Additionally, blind babies often seem not to be emotionally bonded or attached to their mothers. However, research seems to indicate that the insufficiency of stimuli in tactile, kinesthetic, and auditory areas in the early years of life is as much a factor in the bizarre behavior of these children as is the blindness per se. Appropriate stimulation in these modes facilitates the development of normal attachment to the mother. Similar evidence is available regarding early intervention with the deaf; intervention with deaf children before the age of two often results in their adaptation to normal classrooms, whereas deaf children who are not in intervention programs until after three years of age frequently fail to make such adaptations.

Early intervention by means of physical therapy for the young child with cerebral palsy is finally receiving the attention in this country that it has had in European medical centers for many years. Early identification of infants under one year of age who are developing cerebral palsy is occurring in clinics that closely follow high risk groups, such as premature infants. Evidence of improved quality of motor development following early and regular physical therapy is accumulating, and—probably most important of all, but not measured by most research projects—parents consistently report benefits in their handling and feeding of, and overall interaction with, these difficult-to-manage infants.

This chapter has thus far focused on fairly distinct and identifiable clinical conditions in which the rationale for early intervention is probably recognized and accepted by the majority of physicians who care for young children. We shall now turn to the far more commonly encountered clinical problem of what physicians can advise parents of young children with severe or mild, generalized or specific, developmental delays to do for their children. Is there a rational basis for early intervention with these children as an alternate approach to previously mentioned attitudes of hopelessness or false reassurance?

TWO MAJOR TYPES OF MENTAL RETARDATION

Mental (or developmental) retardation refers to significantly subaverage general intellectual functioning existing concurrently with deficits in adaptive behavior and manifested during the developmental period. It is not a single disease syndrome or symptom; it rather is a state of impairment which is recognized in the behavior of the individual. Most often the specific etiology is unknown.

It is useful to subdivide mental retardation into two broad categories: severe involvement (biological) and mild involvement (cultural-familial). Children with severe involvement have I.Q. scores of less than 50, and frequently manifest overt brain damage as a cause. Severe developmental retardation is distributed equally across all social classes and does not generally cluster in families. In contrast, children with mild involvement have I.Q. scores in the 50 to 70 range, and seldom manifest obvious signs of brain damage. Mild developmental retardation is predominantly found in the lower social classes and has a strong familial incidence. Etiologically, environmental factors are felt to be very important in mild retardation and less so in severe retardation. An overwhelming number of retarded children are mildly involved (89 percent), with about 11 percent severely involved. Thus, there would seem to be a real potential to alter the course and improve the outlook for many mildly delayed young children. Furthermore, it is becoming increasingly clear that the ultimate prognosis for retarded children depends more on factors such as social adaptation, motivation, educational opportunities, and vocational skills than on I.Q. scores alone.

TWO OPPOSING THEORIES OF INTELLECTUAL DEVELOPMENT

When deciding how to treat developmentally retarded children, the physician often runs directly into the eternal nature vs. nurture controversy. Some investigators believe that intellectual development is primarily affected by the environment ("nurture"); others claim that development is largely predetermined by heredity ("nature").

Arthur R. Jensen of the University of California, a prominent spokesman for genetic determinism, thinks the environment functions as a threshold variable. By this, he means that a certain minimal quality of environment is necessary for normal intellectual development; he believes that above this threshold, variations in the environment do not cause major differences in intelligence.

In sharp contrast is Dr. Benjamin S. Bloom of the University of Chicago, who envisions environmental variations as a continuum from good to bad, with the quality of the environment having a linear relationship to the development of intelligence. The more abundant the environment, the closer an individual comes to performing at the level set by his or her biological limits; the more deprived the environment, the greater the extent to which intelligence is depressed. An important corollary of Bloom's theory is that intelligence develops most rapidly during the first few years of life. He finds that about 50 percent of I.Q. differences at maturity can be explained by I.Q. differences at age four. Thus, when considering intellectual development, environmental intervention has the greatest impact if it is provided during the early preschool years, before a child is four years of age.

Bloom's conclusions are frequently cited as the rationale for early intervention. Dr. Burton White of Harvard University recently supported this viewpoint when he wrote: "After 17 years of research on how human beings acquire their abilities, I have become convinced that it is to the first three years of life that we should now turn most of our attention. My own studies, as well as the work of many others, have clearly indicated that the experiences of those first years are far more important than we had previously thought. In their simple everyday activities, infants and toddlers form the foundations of all later development."

INTERVENTION PROGRAMS LESS WELL-ACCEPTED BY PHYSICIANS

From this theoretical background in the mid-1960s grew two major types of early stimulation/education programs. One type, exemplified by Project Head Start, focused on children of low-income families who constituted a high risk group for cultural-familial retardation. The goal of this type of program is to prevent the borderline mental retardation and school failure attributable to environments that fail to adequately support development. The other type of program was directed at infants and children with recognized early developmental delays, such as Down Syndrome, generalized psychomotor retardation, infantile autism, or specific language delay. The goal of this type of program is to maximize the developmental potential of the biologically impaired child, and to prevent the phenomenon of secondary environmental deprivation which can occur even in well-intentioned homes.

Does early intervention work? Dr. Alice Hayden of the University of Washington, a long-time leader in this field, recently wrote: "No one involved in early intervention escapes asking himself why one ought to engage in such an effort, if only because the question is asked of us so often by others. Self-questioning inevitably follows questioning by parents, physicians, legislators, and colleagues in the field." Researchers have learned that this is a complex question which must be answered on several different levels. The major proof of effectiveness most commonly sought is permanent gains in I.Q. scores by children in special intervention programs. This variable is the easiest to measure and the "flashiest" with which to advertise results. Unfortunately, it is probably a very poor index of the ways in which children benefit from early intervention. Much of the early pessimism and skepticism surrounding early intervention efforts was due to the fact that follow-up research was not showing significant and long-lasting I.Q. gains for children in special programs.

However, recent work focusing on harder-to-measure outcome variables is documenting program effectiveness in areas with more functional significance than simple I.Q. scores. Many programs for children from low socioeconomic homes are finding long-range gains in academic achievement with reduction in grade failures and less need for special education services. This is especially true for programs that start early in a child's life and actively involve parents. Programs for developmentally delayed children are enhancing specific deficit areas, such as language, and are teaching specific coping skills and behaviors. Children with Down Syndrome are reading, dancing, and participating in the full range of preschool activities; children with marked language delays are participating in group story-telling and learning previously-absent social skills. Preliminary data indicates that school-age children with Down Syndrome who received special education as infants or young children are performing better than Down Syndrome children who received no early intervention. Gains by program children in the area of personal-social behaviors, such as feeding, washing, and dressing, have been consistently found. Certainly of equal importance, most of these programs provide parent support, counseling, and relief, with consequently improved family functioning.

BASES FOR EARLY INTERVENTION

Considering all recent information, rational bases for early developmental intervention include the following eight points.

1. Early experience influences all areas of development. Indeed, all current research leads to the conclusion that the development of any human ability results from a complex, dynamic interaction of both genetic and environmental factors. Someone has said that the appropriate answer to the age-old question, "Which is more important?" is, "It is 100 percent nature and 100 percent nurture." The main difference is that physicians have some potential ability to positively influence the "nurture" part.

2. Several long-term studies indicate that the outcome for children who have experienced perinatal distress is greatly determined by their subsequent environmental experiences. Various longitudinal studies of prenatal and perinatal complications have yet to produce a single predictive variable more potent than the familial and socioeconomic characteristics of the caretaking environment. The effects of social class tended to reduce or amplify intellectual deficits. In advantaged families, infants who had suffered perinatal complications such as prematurity, anoxia, or asymptomatic intrauterine infection generally showed no significant (or only small) residual effects on follow-up. Many infants from disadvantaged homes with identical histories of complications showed significant retardation in later functioning.

3. Research has shown that there may be critical periods for the development of

certain skills, and that most of these periods may occur during the first four years of life. Bloom's theory of how intelligence develops places great emphasis on the period of infancy and early childhood when the rate of brain growth and central nervous system maturation is maximal.

4. Failure to provide a stimulating early environment leads not only to a continuation of the developmental status quo, but to actual atrophy of sensory abilities and to developmental regression. It is known that early visual deprivation caused by strabismus can lead to atrophy of visual structures with loss of function, and it appears that early auditory deprivation caused by chronic otitis media may have a similar effect on auditory structures and function. Developmentally delayed children are at particular risk for secondary deprivation when even "good" environments "turn off" because of lack of expected feedback. Thus, a major role of early intervention is to maximize—not normalize—a child's developmental rate, even if that optimal biologic rate is significantly less than the norm.

5. Failure to remediate one handicap may multiply its effects in other developmental areas, and may produce social and emotional handicaps that are secondary to the initial insult. It has been found that a handicap in one sensory system will often produce handicaps in another system. Thus, when the "sensory synergism" which one system ordinarily provides for another breaks down, the effect of the original handicap is multiplied. When hearing is deprived in early life, visual perception is disturbed and vice-versa. Here again the strong possibility of compounding a handicap exists, for parents of an unresponsive, hearing-impaired infant may perceive the child as rejecting and dull if they are unaware of the disability. Thus, a vicious cycle can be set up in which the very handicap the child is born with leads to less effective care-giving.

6. When recognition of an intellectual or cognitive handicap is delayed, the child's developmental status inevitably becomes worse with respect to other children over time. It has been shown that a handicapped child entering school ranking only one standard deviation below the mean in I.Q. or other tests of ability will tend to rank even lower by adolescence. Part of the reason for this progressive deterioration in a child's relative developmental standing may be that the fact of a handicap tends to alter the responses of parents, teachers, and other caregivers in the environment. This problem has been demonstrated in several studies of children with Down Syndrome.

7. Early intervention can work to reduce and ameliorate the effects of a handicapping condition, and can do so more surely and rapidly than later intervention. Professionals in the field must stop evaluating early intervention on the basis of dramatic cures, such as I.Q. gains, and concentrate instead on modifying the course of handicapping conditions. Adequate research evidence exists in support of the ability of early intervention to positively influence the day-to-day functioning of handicapped children. Several longitudinal studies are now indicating that up to one-third of these children are able to enter regular classes; in these classrooms they are keeping pace with their regular education peers and are not repeating grades.

8. Parents need models of good parenting behavior with a handicapped child and specific instructions for working with their child in a naturally stimulating manner. The parents of a handicapped child are often worn down by shock, grief, and sheer physical fatigue, and they very much need direction from a trained professional. Early intervention can support parents in their grief and relative helplessness, and can model a positive interventionist role for them to assume in working with their child. It can also provide the relief many parents need to re-establish normal relationships with their spouse and other children in the family.

SUMMARY

Does early intervention work? Yes. It works to improve the prognosis for developmentally disabled children and their families. Just as it is an integral part of the physician's role to manage and care for children with incurable physical diseases like cancer, cystic fibrosis, and inoperable congenital heart disease, so it is equally important for the physician to be a leader and advocate for children with mental and developmental disorders.

Is the research data clear-cut about the effects of early intervention? Not at all. Ideally, we would know much more about the precise variables that account for the success of early intervention in some cases and its failure to produce results in others. We would know more about possible harmful effects of too much early intervention in overstimulating the handicapped child and the child's family. Dr. Jerome Kagan of Harvard University aptly summarizes the state of the art: "The recent crest of interest in developmental psychology has produced a *tiny* corpus of *moderately firm* facts that invite reexamination of the presuppositions that have guided so much past work."

However, we cannot afford to wait until all the research results are in to begin applying what is known. Handicapped patients and their parents will no longer tolerate this approach. Nearly all the dramatic progress in the area of developmental disabilities over the past 20 years has occurred not because of the leadership and direction of physicians, psychologists, educators, or legislators, but because of the dedicated efforts of parents working together. We do know enough already to reject the two popular misconceptions mentioned at the beginning of this lesson: (1) that nothing useful can be done for severely impaired children; and (2) that most mildly delayed children will eventually outgrow their problems. We do know enough already to strongly encourage primary care physicians of young children to make early identification and intervention for developmental problems an integral part of day-to-day practice.

BIBLIOGRAPHY

Caldwell, B. M., and Stedman, D. J. *Infant education: A guide for helping handicapped children in the first three years.* New York: Walker, 1977.

Haskins, R., Finkelstein, N. W., and Stedman, D. J. Infant-stimulation programs and their effects. *Pediatric Annals*, 1978, *7*, 123–146.

Hayden, A. H., and McGinness, G. D. Bases for early intervention. In E. Sontag (Ed.), *Educational programming for the severely and profoundly handicapped.* Reston, Va.: CECMR, 1977.

Hayden, A. H., Morris, K., and Barley, D. *The effectiveness of early education for handicapped children: Final report.* Seattle: University of Washington, 1977.

MacMillan, D. L. *Mental retardation in school and society.* Boston: Little, Brown, and Co., 1977.

Marquis, P. Cognitive stimulation. *American Journal of Diseases of Children*, 1976, *130*, 410–415.

Sameroff, A., and Chandler, M. Infant casualty and the continuum of infant caretaking. In F. D. Horowitz, E. M. Hetherington, M. Siegel, and S. Scarr-Salapatek (Eds.), *Review of child development research* (Vol. 4) Chicago: University of Chicago Press, 1975.

Werner, E. E., Bierman, J. M., and French, F. E. *The children of Kauai.* Honolulu: University of Hawaii Press, 1971.

White, B. L. *The first three years of life.* Englewood Cliffs, N.J.: Prentice-Hall, Inc., 1975.

Chapter 3

Goal

To develop skills in screening children with the Denver Developmental Screening Test (DDST) and the Denver Prescreening Developmental Questionnaire (PDQ).

Objectives

At the end of this chapter, the physician should be able to:
- explain the rationale for routinely screening all children for development;
- discuss the appropriate use of the DDST in clinical practice;
- discuss the appropriate use of the PDQ in clinical practice.

DEVELOPMENTAL SCREENING

By
WILLIAM K. FRANKENBURG, M.D.,
ALMA W. FANDAL, and
MELINDA B. KEMPER, M.A.

I. Rationale for Routine Developmental Screening
   A. Earlier intervention offers hope of more effective treatment and better prognosis.
   B. Developmental disabilities are very common in young children and can affect growth and abilities throughout the child's life.
   C. Commonly used techniques for identification—including developmental history, clinical judgment, and informal observation of developmental milestones and language ability—are inaccurate methods of detecting children with possible developmental handicaps.
II. Developmental Screening Instruments
   A. The Denver Developmental Screening Test (DDST) was developed to provide a simple-to-administer yet highly accurate and reliable method of identifying developmentally delayed children.
   B. In the two-stage screening process, the Prescreening Developmental Questionnaire (PDQ) can be used by physicians serving parents who have at least completed high school, and the short form of the DDST can be used by physicians serving parents with less than a high school education.
   C. All children should be screened at the following ages: three to six months; nine to 12 months; 18 to 24 months; and at three, four, and five years of age.
III. The Denver Developmental Screening Test
   A. The DDST is highly accurate in identifying infants and children with developmental disorders.
   B. The DDST consists of a kit of materials, a score sheet, and a reference manual.
   C. The 105 items on the test form are arranged in developmental sequence in four major areas: personal-social, fine motor-adaptive, language, and gross motor.
   D. The child's ability to perform 25 to 30 tasks results in a test score which is "normal," "abnormal," "questionable," or "untestable."
IV. The Denver Developmental Screening Test-Short Form
   A. Administration of the short form is similar to that of the full DDST.
   B. Only the 12 items mastered by 90 percent of children the same age as the child being tested are used.
   C. If a child fails or refuses one of the 12 items, the short DDST is considered suspect and the full DDST is administered while the child is in the test setting; approximately 25 percent of children screened with the short DDST will require rescreening with the full DDST.
V. The Prescreening Developmental Questionnaire
   A. The PDQ was formulated from questions on the DDST.
   B. There are five steps in administering the PDQ:

     1. Calculating the child's age;
     2. Marking 10 age-appropriate questions on the test form;
     3. Instructing the parents to read the directions and answer all 10 questions;
     4. Checking to see that the parents followed the instructions;
     5. Determining the child's total test score.
  C. A score of nine or 10 is not suspect, while a score of eight or below would require rescreening with the PDQ in two to four weeks
VI. Summary

RATIONALE FOR ROUTINE DEVELOPMENTAL SCREENING

The importance of preventing developmental handicaps such as mental retardation is well accepted. Such prevention has generally taken two approaches. The first is primary prevention, which involves total prevention of the problem through such efforts as genetic counseling, better pre- and perinatal care, immunization against such diseases as measles, and improvement of the social environment of those children who are at risk. The secondary form of prevention consists of early identification of children with developmental handicaps either to reverse or to ameliorate the problem and thereby improve the long-term prognosis. It is well known that developmental handicaps are secondary to a variety of biological and environmental factors. Therefore, in general, the earlier intervention is begun, the better the prognosis and the more cost-effective the treatment.

Because physicians caring for infants and preschool-age children have frequent contact with the children and their families during the first six years of life, they are in a strategic position to identify handicaps as soon as such deviations arise. Thus, physicians can help promote the secondary prevention of developmental handicaps.

There is no longer any question about whether or not physicians should assume this identification role. The American Academy of Pediatrics' Standards of Child Health Care has consistently stressed such a role as one essential component of well child health care. Furthermore, a recent nationwide survey of the American Academy of Pediatrics has demonstrated that growth and development problems are some of the most common childhood disorders encountered by physicians who care for infants and preschool-age children.

Not only is routine screening essential to good health care, but the early identification of developmental deviations is one of the most productive activities a physician can undertake. Developmental problems, which are among the most common disorders for which screening is done, require early treatment in order to be most effective.

Surveys of pediatricians from 1964 to 1974 in Great Britain and the United States have shown that physicians generally rely on the following methods of identifying developmental handicaps: (1) obtaining a past history of developmental landmarks; (2) making a clinical judgment which relies on a so-called response to the clinical situation; (3) observing a few motor developmental landmarks; and later, (4) observing speech and language ability. Various studies have consistently demonstrated these approaches to be insufficient, since past recall of developmental landmarks is grossly inaccurate and major milestones of achievement such as sitting, standing, and walking may be normal in 50 percent of retarded children. In a study by Bierman (1964) of 681 two-year-olds, pediatricians correctly identified only three out of 11 retarded children. In another study by Korsch (1961), it was noted that pediatricians consistently overrated the I.Q.s of retarded children. In other words, the physicians failed to identify the retarded.

These errors in clinical judgment were not related to the age of the child or the physician's knowledge of the child through frequent contacts. Likewise, the physician's years of experience and level of confidence were not relevant factors. Nor, it should be noted, were some physicians much more accurate than others.

The findings of these studies are 10 years old. Today, it might be expected that the situation had changed, since developmental screening is taught in most pediatric training programs. However, it is disturbing to find a recent survey indicating that only 10 percent of pediatricians actually screened all children for developmental problems.

The chief reason physicians gave for failing to screen all of their patients was lack of time. This situation is alarming, since the professional and lay public have relied upon physicians to identify the majority of developmentally delayed children as early as possible. Yet the physicians are not identifying these children, due to the reliance upon inaccurate methods of assessment. Since the majority of developmentally handicapped children are still not identified until they fail in school, there has been a recent trend for schools to launch their own large-scale early identification programs among infants and preschool-age children.

DEVELOPMENTAL SCREENING INSTRUMENTS

A number of years ago, concerns about the inadequacy of commonly-used screening techniques led to the development of the Denver Developmental Screening Test (DDST). The DDST has been demonstrated to be simple to administer and acceptable to the public, as well as reliable and accurate in identifying developmentally delayed children.

Because physicians needed something quick that could be routinely administered to all children at periodic intervals, a two-stage screening procedure was developed. In this two-stage process, all children periodically undergo the quick first-stage screen. Only those who are suspect are screened further with the second stage of the test. Those who are again suspect on the second screen should receive a complete diagnostic evaluation as soon as possible.

Originally, it was envisioned that the Denver Prescreening Developmental Questionnaire (PDQ), which is a parent-answered questionnaire, would serve as a first-stage screen and the DDST as a second. However, a recent study compared the use of the PDQ and DDST among 10,000 children screened in private pediatricians' offices and in public health clinics.

The private pediatricians' offices primarily served parents who had completed some education beyond high school; the clinics primarily serviced parents who had a high school education or less. The study revealed that the most cost-efficient method of screening children of better-educated parents was to use the PDQ as the first stage screen, and to follow-up suspect children with a second PDQ. However, in the case of the clinic practices servicing the less educated parents, using a short form of the DDST as the first stage screen and the full DDST for the suspect cases was found to be best in identifying the retarded.

It is recommended that all children undergo a first stage screen (either the PDQ or shortened DDST) at the following ages: three to six months; nine to 12 months; 18 to 24 months; and again at three, four, and five years of age. By screening at these ages, the physician should be able to identify the majority of children with problems early enough to facilitate effective intervention.

THE DENVER DEVELOPMENTAL SCREENING TEST

Various studies have demonstrated that the DDST effectively identifies between 85 and 100 percent of the infants and preschool-age children who are developmentally retarded. Follow-up has shown that at least 89 percent of those children who had abnormal DDST results were failing in school five to six years later, indicating that few children outgrow early developmental delays.

Busy pediatric health care facilities, however, do not use the DDST for the routine screening it was designed to encourage. Although many physicians have been introduced to the test in medical school and most acknowledge the importance of routine developmental screening, physicians' use of the DDST is often restricted to confirming suspicions of a developmental delay. The reason most often given for this restricted use is that there is simply not enough time to administer a 15- to 20-minute test to all children who are seen at the recommended ages.

A shortened version of the DDST was developed which reduces the time required to only five to 10 minutes and yet identifies as suspect those children who are likely to have abnormal, questionable, or untestable scores when given a full DDST. Since accurate administration of the shortened test is dependent upon knowledge of the full DDST, a brief overview of the full test is necessary. Following this overview is a discussion of the short DDST.

The DDST is a reliable, economic screening device for detecting children who have a high probability of being developmentally impaired. It is valuable for screening asymptomatic children for possible developmental problems and for confirming intuitive suspicions of delay with an objective measure. The DDST is also an effective instrument for monitoring high risk children such as those who have experienced perinatal difficulties.

A few points should be emphasized, however, in order to insure proper usage of the DDST:

1. It is a screening test—not an I.Q. test and not a definitive predictor of current or future adaptive or intellectual ability.
2. It alerts the professional to possible problems. It does not generate diagnostic labels such as learning disability, language disorder, or emotional disturbance. It should never

be substituted for a diagnostic evaluation or physical examination.
3. In order to be valid, it *must* be administered in the standardized manner with exact test materials.

The test consists of a kit of inexpensive materials, a score sheet, and a reference manual. Probably the most important element in the proper administration of the DDST is the reference manual which contains instructions for calculating the child's age and making necessary adjustments for prematurity. The manual also explains the formula for interpreting total results and gives precise instructions for administration and interpretation of each item. It contains a checklist to enable the tester to make sure the correct testing procedures have been followed, and a helpful bibliography of published books and articles about the DDST.

The DDST is given to well children—or those who are apparently well—to sort out children who have a high probability of being developmentally impaired. Administration of the test requires about 15 to 20 minutes. Designed for use with children from birth to six years of age, the DDST is given by asking the child to perform various tasks appropriate for his or her age. If the child does not perform the selected tasks, the examiner is alerted to the fact that this child may have a problem and will need a more comprehensive evaluation.

The DDST, which was standardized on a cross-sectional sample of Denver children, can be accurately applied to all racial groups. It provides not only a valid, concrete method for measuring a child's performance against a standardization sample, but also a one-page profile of the child's progress during the preschool years.

On the DDST form, there are 105 tasks that most children perform before the age of six years. These tasks were selected from existing infant and preschool scales on the basis of their validity, ease of administration, and clarity of scoring. For example, one task on the form is "walks well." This task, like all others on the test, represents skills that are acquired by different children at different ages. One child might begin walking at 10 months; another perfectly normal child may not walk until 14 months. This range could be represented, as in Figure 3-1, on a cumulative frequency curve.

Because this type of graph would be cumbersome on a test form, the information on the graph was condensed into a bar on Figure 3-2. This bar graph is placed on the DDST form in relation to the age lines at the top and bottom of the form. The left end of the bar corresponds to the age when 25 percent of the children normally perform the item. The hatchmark indicates when 50 percent perform the task; the left end of the colored shading marks when 75 percent perform it; and the right end of the bar indicates when 90 percent of the children normally perform the task.

On the DDST (see Figure 3-3), the tasks are arranged in developmental sequence. For example, the majority of children perform the task "walks backwards" at a later age than "walks well." Therefore, the bar is placed on the age line slightly to the right of the "walks well" task, as can be seen in the gross motor sector.

The 105 tasks on the DDST are arranged under four major headings. Those tasks measuring self-help skills and ability to get along with people are in the personal-social section. The second section, fine motor-adaptive, measures the child's ability to perceive, use his or her hands, pick up objects, and draw. Those tasks which measure language—the child's ability to respond to sound, follow instructions, and speak—are presented in the language section. And finally, tasks relating to locomotion and body posture are presented in the gross-motor section.

In administering the DDST, it is not necessary to ask the child to perform all of the test items. Instead, a vertical line is drawn on the form at the exact age of the child (calculated according to instructions in the reference manual). This line, cutting through all four sections of the test, helps determine which tasks the child should be asked to perform. It is usually only necessary to administer about 25 or 30 items for each child.

In administering the test, the examiner seeks to determine whether or not the child can perform tasks that a normal child of that age can perform. Responses must be interpreted in strict accordance with guidelines given in the reference manual so that the child's performance can be correctly evaluated and compared with that of the standardization sample.

Some items are passed by observing the child perform the tasks. Others, such as whether or not the child can dress himself or herself, may be scored upon report of the parent. As the child passes or fails an item, a "P" or "F" is placed on the bar.

After each item has been scored, the next step is to identify delays. Inability to perform any item which falls completely to the left of the age line should be considered a delay. In other words, 90 percent of normal children can pass that item at a younger age than the age of the child being tested. Failure to perform an item which touches the vertical age line is not considered to be a delay.

The number of delays and their location within the sectors are important in determining a total test result of normal, abnormal, questionable, or untestable. A formula given in the reference manual is used to determine the child's overall score. Abnormal, questionable, or untestable scores are considered to be positive test results. Approximately 10 percent of the children between birth and six years of age will receive positive test results. Determining why the result is positive and what should be done about it are two of the major responsibilities of the physician and other professionals serving the child.

Although the professional health provider must know the test in order to interpret it to parents and to follow-up on a positive test result, it is not necessary that the test be administered only by a physician. In many instances specially trained technicians and aides administer the test, and the professional interprets it and provides follow-up.

The question often arises as to whether or not the physician needs to know how to administer the test even though he or she does not routinely administer it in practice. When asked about this, most physicians agree that unless

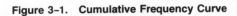

Figure 3–1.   Cumulative Frequency Curve

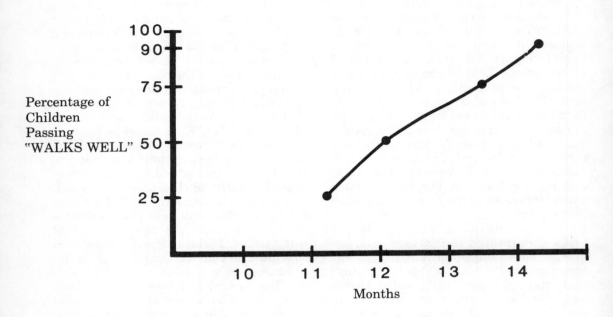

Figure 3–2.   Cumulative Frequency Bar Graph

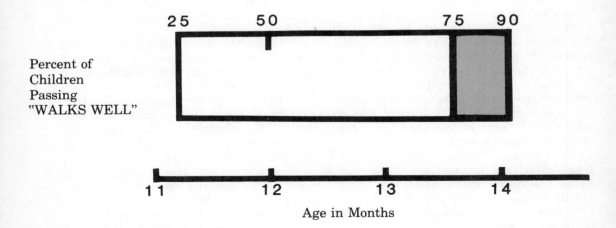

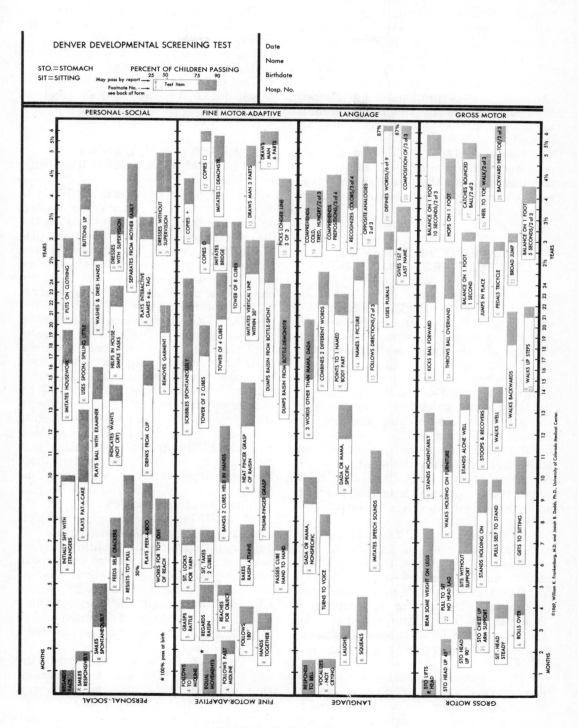

Figure 3-3. Sample DDST

one has had the experiences of actually testing a number of children, it is practically impossible to adequately supervise, interpret, and follow-up DDST results.

In order to use the DDST properly, a potential examiner should study the test manual, view the demonstration film, and complete the proficiency evaluation. Without carefully studying these training materials, professionals and paraprofessionals alike will not be able to administer a valid test. If the items are not administered and interpreted in the standardized manner, the test may only represent a subjective interpretation by an individual examiner.

DENVER DEVELOPMENTAL SCREENING TEST-SHORT FORM

Once an examiner is proficient in administering the DDST, applying the short method is quite simple. Preparation of the form requires the same careful calculation of a child's age and placement of the age line, but only 12 items need to be administered for the shortened form. As shown in Figure 3-4 (see following page), the three items which are immediately to the left of, but not touching, the age line in each of the four sections are administered. If all 12 items are passed, this first stage screening with the short DDST is considered non-suspect, and the child would receive no further testing until he or she reaches the next age on the periodic screening schedule.

If, however, one of 12 items is refused or is failed, as in the personal-social sector shown in Figure 3-4, the short DDST result would be considered suspect and a full DDST should be completed while the child is in the test setting. Approximately 25 percent of the children screened with the short DDST will receive suspect scores and will need to be given the full DDST.

This method of two-stage screening is recommended for use in offices where the educational level of the parents served is likely to be less than high school. In settings where staff time prohibits the use of the full DDST for all children, the short DDST prescreen has several advantages:

1. It saves time.
2. There is only one result to be reported to the parents and entered in the child's record.
3. There is no time lapse between the first and second stage of screening.
4. The child does not have to be rescheduled for the second level of screening.

THE PRESCREENING DEVELOPMENTAL QUESTIONNAIRE

In offices where parents are likely to have a high school education or better, developmental screening can rely on the use of a parent-answered questionnaire. While parents may not remember key points in their child's developmental history, studies have shown that they can report the child's current achievements quite accurately.

The PDQ was developed by formulating questions from DDST items. A receptionist or office assistant can prepare a PDQ for a child in only a minute or two, and parents can complete the PDQ while waiting to see the physician. The PDQ, an easy-to-administer test, can be incorporated into the routine for each well child check-up, even in the busiest offices. Also, since the PDQ requires only minimal participation by the child, it is a useful tool for screening children who may be brought to the physician's office because of illness or other problems.

The PDQ (a scored sample of which is included as Figure 3-5) consists of 97 questions that focus on a child's current behavior. These questions are arranged in chronological order according to the age at which 90 percent of the DDST normative sample passed the corresponding DDST item. Questions are printed on five color-coded forms and cover the ages from three months to six years.

There are five steps to administering and scoring the PDQ, and it is important that each of these steps be performed carefully and accurately. Since it is expected that physicians will be able to administer the PDQ after studying this lesson, these five steps will be described in detail below.

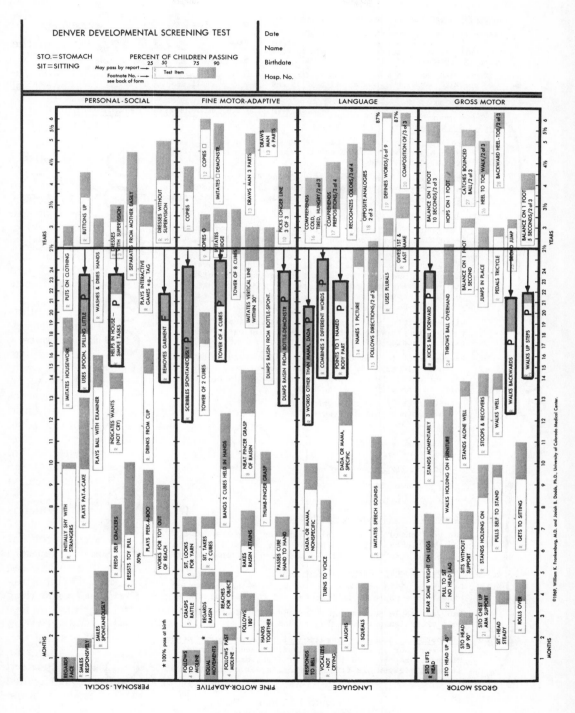

Figure 3–4. DDST Short Form

4 year

DENVER PRESCREENING DEVELOPMENTAL QUESTIONNAIRE

Please read each question carefully before you answer. Circle the best answer for each question. YOUR CHILD IS NOT EXPECTED TO BE ABLE TO DO EVERYTHING THE QUESTIONS ASK.

Child's Name Ronald Jones

Date 5/28/76

Birthdate 5/20/72

YES – CHILD CAN DO NOW or HAS DONE IN THE PAST
NO – CHILD CANNOT DO NOW, HAS NOT DONE IN THE PAST or YOU ARE NOT SURE THAT YOUR CHILD CAN DO IT.

R   – CHILD REFUSES TO TRY
NO-OPP – CHILD HAS NOT HAD THE CHANCE TO TRY

© Wm. K. Frankenburg, M.D., University of Colorado Medical Center, 1975.

4 year check – Answer 71 through 80

9

71. Can your child pedal a tricycle at least ten feet? If your child has never had a chance to ride a tricycle his size, circle NO-OPP. (YES) NO R NO-OPP

72. After eating, does your child wash and dry his hands well enough so you don't have to do them over? Circle NO-OPP if you do not allow him to wash and dry his hands by himself. (YES) NO R NO-OPP

4 year, 3 month check – Answer 73 through 82

73. Does your child put an "s" at the end of his words when he is talking about more than one thing such as block<u>s</u>, shoe<u>s</u> or toy<u>s</u>? (YES) NO R NO-OPP

74. Without letting your child hold onto anything, have him balance on one foot for as long as he can. Encourage him by showing him how, if necessary. GIVE HIM THREE CHANCES. Estimate seconds by counting slowly. Did your child balance 2 seconds or more? (YES) NO R NO-OPP

75. Without letting your child take a running jump, ask him to jump length-wise over this paper. Did he do this without landing on the paper? (YES) NO R NO-OPP

76. Have your child draw this figure in the space below. DO NOT SAY "CIRCLE". <u>Do not help or correct your child</u>. Say to your child, "Draw a picture just like this one", and point to the picture on the right.

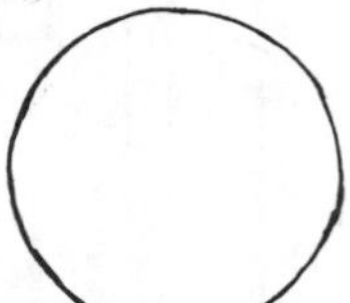

   Look at these examples when scoring your child's drawing.

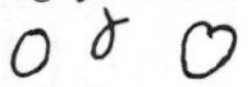

   Answer YES

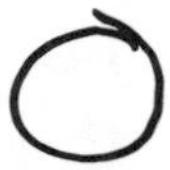

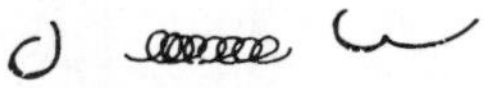

   Answer NO

   Did your child draw a circle? (YES) NO R NO-OPP

4 year, 6 month check – Answer 77 through 86

77. Can your child put <u>eight</u> blocks on top of one another without the blocks falling? This applies to <u>small</u> blocks about 1 inch in size and not blocks more than 2 inches in size. (YES) NO R NO-OPP

4 year, 9 month check – Answer 78 through 87

78. Does your child play hide-and-seek, cops-and-robbers or other games where he takes turns and follows rules? (YES) NO R NO-OPP

79. Can your child put jeans, shirt, dress or socks on without help except snapping, buttoning and belts? YES (NO) R NO-OPP

80. <u>Without your coaching or saying his name so he can repeat it</u>, does your child say both his first and last name? Nicknames may be used in place of first name. Circle NO if he only gives his first name or is not easily understood. (YES) NO R NO-OPP

5/28/76

Figure 3-5 Sample PDQ

Step 1. The child's age must be precisely calculated to the nearest month so that the correct questions may be assigned. This step is critically important, because if a child's age is not correctly calculated, the appropriate questions cannot be assigned, and the PDQ results will be invalid. To calculate a child's age, the child's birthdate (written as the year, then the month, then the day) is subtracted from the date the test is given.

For example, if a child who was born on August 25, 1974, were to be tested on January 10, 1979, the calculation of exact age would be as follows:

```
  79-1-10    (test date: January 10, 1979)
− 74-8-25    (birthdate: August 25, 1974)
   4-4-15    (exact age: 4 years, 4 months,
             and 15 days)
```

In subtracting, if it becomes necessary to borrow days from the month column, a month is considered to have 30 days. Likewise a year is written as 12 months.

For purposes of the PDQ, the child's age is rounded off to the nearest month. Fifteen days or fewer are considered to be less than a month; more than 15 days are counted as a whole month. Thus, in the example above, the child is considered to be four years and four months old.

Step 2. After determining the child's age, it is necessary to select 10 age-appropriate questions. Printed in the upper left corner of each side of the five color-coded forms are the ages covered on that page. To assign the 10 age-appropriate questions, it is necessary to select the age on the form which is closest to the age calculated. For the four-year-four-month-old child, the closest age on the forms would be four years and three months, which includes questions 73 through 82. The examiner would mark these questions with brackets, give the form to the parent, and ask him or her to answer the questions as accurately as possible.

Some receptionists or office assistants prefer to do Steps 1 and 2 before the scheduled office visit. Then the PDQ forms are ready when the parent and child arrive for the appointment.

Step 3. In administering the PDQ, the examiner should instruct the parent to read the directions at the top of the PDQ form and to answer each of the 10 bracketed questions by circling "yes," "no," "refuses," or "no opportunity." Some of the PDQ questions require the parent to ask the child to perform a task, such as copy a circle or hop on one foot. The PDQ tells the parent exactly how to administer the item and what constitutes a passing performance.

Step 4. After the parent has completed the questionnaire, the examiner must check to see that all 10 of the bracketed questions have been answered. If a parent has failed to answer any of the questions, the PDQ is returned to the parent to be completed.

Step 5. After the test has been completed, it is necessary to count the "yes" answers to get a total score. It is recommended that PDQ scores of nine or 10 "yesses" be considered nonsuspect. Scores of eight or fewer should be considered suspect and would require rescreening with the PDQ two to four weeks later. When rescreening with the PDQ, the examiner must again calculate the child's age since the child will be older and may require different questions. A child who receives a score of six or fewer "yesses" on the second PDQ should be referred for diagnostic testing. A child who receives a score of more than six on the second PDQ would receive no further testing until he or she reaches the next age on the periodic screening schedule.

Research has indicated that the above PDQ cut-off scores will identify all children who are significantly delayed in development and a large number of children with borderline delays. Children with persistent borderline delays who are missed on initial screening can be identified with periodic rescreening. The recommended cut-off scores will identify the maximum number of children with developmental disorders without generating unacceptable overreferral rates. However, non-suspect screening results are not a guarantee of problem-free development. If the physician or the parents are concerned about some aspect of a child's development, that child should receive further testing, regardless of the PDQ score.

Studies using the PDQ have shown that very few children with I.Q.s between 52 and 83, and less than half with I.Q.s less than 52 had been previously identified. In one case, for example, a 15-month-old child who had had 12 well child check-ups was identified as suspect by a PDQ given during the 13th check-up. On further testing, he demonstrated delays in many areas, especially in cognition and language (DQ: <68). This case is not atypical. Children with delayed gross motor development (with or without abnormal neurological findings) were no more likely to have been previously identified.

In research on the PDQ, private practitioners screened over 5,000 children by using this instrument. Obviously this would not have been possible without widespread lay and professional acceptance. Parents like the PDQ because it gives them something interesting to do while waiting for the physician. They are curious about their children's abilities and welcome the opportunity to see if their children are doing as well as they should be. Also, developmental screening indicates to parents that the physician really cares about the child's total development. Physicians like the PDQ because it provides a quick, simple, and economical method of identifying children who need further testing as well as a convenient method of assessing a child's development.

SUMMARY

Primary care physicians are responsible for the early identification of children with developmental problems. Physicians should routinely and periodically screen the development of all children with standard screening tests of proven accuracy. The recommended ages for screening are three to six, nine to 12, and 18 to 24 months, and three, four, and five years of age.

To facilitate such routine mass screening, a two-stage screening process consisting of the following can be used:

1. the short and full DDST for health programs serving children whose parents have primarily less than a high school education;
2. the PDQ for health programs serving children whose parents have a high school education or more;
3. the DDST for children whose parents are primarily a mix of educational levels (or if the physician is in doubt which to use).

Before using the DDST, an examiner should first take the prescribed training program and pass the proficiency test. The instructions provided in this chapter should enable a test administrator to use the PDQ.*

A child who is suspect on both of the two stages of the screening process should receive a diagnostic evaluation as soon as possible. Delay in diagnosing and treating handicaps can result in potentially permanent disabilities.

BIBLIOGRAPHY

Bierman, J. M., Connor, A., Vaage, M., and Honzik, M. P. Pediatricians' assessments of the intelligence of two-year-olds and their mental test scores. *Pediatrics,* 1964, *34,* 680–690.

Camp, B. W., van Doorninck, W. J., Frankenburg, W. K., and Lampe, J. M. Preschool developmental testing as a predictor of school problems. *Clinical Pediatrics,* 1977, *16*(3), 257–263.

Frankenburg, W. K., Camp, B. W., De Mersseman, J. A., and Voorhees, S. F. The reliability and stability of the Denver Developmental Screening Test. *Child Development,* 1971, *42,* 1312–1325.

Frankenburg, W. K., Camp, B. W., and VanNatta, P. A. Validity of the Denver Developmental Screening Test. *Child Development,* 1971, *42,* 475–485.

Frankenburg, W. K., and Dodds, J. B. The Denver Developmental Screening Test. *Journal of Pediatrics,* 1967, *71,* 181–191.

Frankenburg, W. K., Dodds, J. B., Fandal, A. W., Kazuk, E., and Cohrs, M. *Denver Developmental*

*DDST materials (including forms, kits, the reference manual, and training films) and PDQ forms can be obtained from: LADOCA Publishing Foundation, East 51st Avenue at Lincoln Street, Denver, Colorado 80216 (telephone 303-629-6379). Other materials distributed by LADOCA include the Denver Articulation Screening Examination, the Denver Eye Screening Test, and the Denver Audiometric Screening Test.

Screening Test: Reference manual. Denver: University of Colorado Medical Center, 1975.

Frankenburg, W. K., Dick, N. P., and Carland, J. Development of preschool aged children of different social and ethnic groups: Implications for developmental screening. *Journal of Pediatrics,* 1975, *87,* 125–132.

Frankenburg, W. K., Goldstein, A., and Camp, B. W. The Revised Denver Developmental Screening Test: Its accuracy as a screening instrument. *Journal of Pediatrics,* 1971, *79,* 988–995.

Frankenburg, W. K., van Doorninck, W. J., Liddell, T. N., and Dick, N. P. The Denver Prescreening Developmental Questionnaire. *Pediatrics,* 1976, *57,* 744–753.

Kemper, M. B., Frankenburg, W. K., Coons, C. E., and Fandal, A. W. *Concurrent validity of a two-stage developmental screening procedure.* Paper presented at meeting of the American Association on Mental Deficiency, Denver, May 1978.

Korsch, B., Cobb, K., and Ashe, B. Pediatricians' appraisals of patients' intelligence. *Pediatrics,* 1961, *27,* 990–1003.

van Doorninck, W. J., Dick, N. P., Frankenburg, W. K., and Liddell, T. N. *Infant and preschool developmental screening and later school performance.* Paper presented at meeting of the Society for Pediatric Research, St. Louis, April 1976.

PART II

Chapter 4

Goal To persuade physicians to take a complete medical history and perform a full physical examination for each child who is suspect on developmental screening.

Objectives At the end of this chapter, the physician should be able to:
- explain how a printed history questionnaire facilitates the taking of a complete developmental history in a minimum amount of time;
- discuss how the questionnaire will facilitate the identification of developmental disorders;
- explain how use of the physical examination form assists the physician in identifying significant etiological factors that may explain the child's developmental problems.

DIAGNOSIS OF SUSPECT AND DELAYED CHILDREN

MEDICAL HISTORY AND PHYSICAL EXAMINATION

By
ROGER V. CADOL, M.D.

I. Introduction
   The complete diagnostic evaluation of a child who is suspected of being developmentally delayed involves compiling a thorough medical history, performing a physical examination, and making other necessary assessments.
II. The Medical History
   A. Developmental deviations may be considered a nonspecific symptom since they can be caused by a variety of factors; thus the history must address each area of potential concern.
   B. The enclosed history form, although quite lengthy, will save a physician's time and the parents' money, and will rule out factors suspected of causing or adding to a child's delay.
III. Case History
   The case involved a three-year-old girl whose severe bilateral sensorineural hearing loss was not discovered when her parents became concerned at one year because the physician assumed he knew the cause of a language delay and did not take a complete history; had a history form been used, treatment for the hearing loss would have been discovered early and the child's prognosis would have been much better.
IV. The Parent Questionnaire
   A. The Parent Questionnaire, which should be completed by the parents at home, will help the physician rule out genetic and congenital disorders, child abuse and neglect, neurological disorders, and vision, hearing, neuromotor, and speech and language problems, and so on.
   B. The physician can explain to parents why their help in filling out the Parent Questionnaire is needed by telling them that the completed questionnaire will help fully understand their child's development.
   C. Because the parents return the questionnaire to the physician prior to meeting with him or her, the physician has time to review the answers and identify items that require further explanation.
   D. The Parent Questionnaire includes a sample Release of Information Form that parents are asked to complete for each professional and facility that has treated or evaluated the child.
   E. Experience with the Parent Questionnaire shows that all parents, even those who have not been privileged to have much education, do complete all or most of the questionnaire; parents see the questionnaire as proof that their physician really cares and has special skills.

V. The Parent Interview
    A. The parent interview should be scheduled when both the physician and the parents can give undivided attention to a discussion of the child's history for an hour; the child should not be present.
    B. The History of the Present Illness form assists in the recording of complete information about the child's current condition by including key words as reminders of important points to be covered.
VI. The Medical Examination
    A. After completion of the parent interview, an appointment should be scheduled to examine the child; the examination is frequently more accurate if the parents prepare the child in advance for the examination.
    B. The enclosed Medical Examination form, like the history, represents a combination of a typical pediatric evaluation with selected additions to identify conditions that may cause the child to be delayed in development.
VII. Summary

INTRODUCTION

A complete diagnostic evaluation of a child who is suspected of being developmentally delayed involves compiling a thorough medical history, performing a physical examination, and making other necessary assessments. The purposes of this chapter are as follows:

1. to explain how the use of a parent-answered history questionnaire enables the physician to take a complete developmental history in a minimum amount of time;
2. to discuss the components of this questionnaire and how it facilitates the identification of developmental disorders;
3. to encourage the physician to make use of the printed history questionnaire form; and
4. to explain how use of the medical examination form assists the physician in identifying significant etiological factors that may explain the child's developmental problems.

THE MEDICAL HISTORY

The accurate diagnosis of developmental disorders relies to a great extent on the physician's thoroughness in taking a child's medical history. An analogy is the diagnosis of neurological disorders which relies extensively upon the history. Developmental deviations may be considered a nonspecific symptom, since they can be caused by a variety of factors—including genetic, neurological, sensory, metabolic, psychiatric, and environmental conditions—and most commonly are caused by a combination of these. Thus, the complete history must address each of these areas of potential concern.

The history form recommended in this chapter is quite lengthy, and no doubt many primary care physicians believe that they cannot spare the time to conduct such history-taking. However, the author believes that use of this form will save time in the long run. Even though the physician may believe that he or she knows the cause of a delay, other factors may be adding to the child's problems. If the physician does not take a detailed history, a factor may be missed which will later necessitate additional visits by the child to the office and the physician may find him- or herself later having to take the portions of the history which earlier were neglected.

CASE HISTORY

Consider the case of a child who was missed because a complete developmental history was not taken by her physician. A three-year-old girl was referred to a developmental diagnostic center when she began to have outbursts of temper directed against her parents and other children. Evaluation at the center showed that she had a severe bilateral sensorineural hearing loss, and that the outbursts were secondary to deafness.

The child's parents had taken the girl to a physician when she was one year old because about that time she stopped babbling and they believed that her speech was not developing properly. Despite the fact that the parents returned to the physician numerous times with their concern, the physician failed to take a complete history.

Instead, he attributed the language delay to two factors. The first was the child's environment; the girl lived in a backwoods area with her parents, who had chosen to "live off the land" at a subsistence level. The physician assumed that these parents were not stimulating the child sufficiently. The second factor was that the girl had a history of recurrent ear infections; the physician assumed that a fluctuating hearing loss associated with otitis media was interfering with the child's development of language.

When the physician became bothered by the child's lack of progress, he reviewed the history more thoroughly, and discovered the child's mother had experienced an undiagnosed fever and rash during the fourth month of pregnancy with the girl. It was later proved that this rash was, in fact, rubella. Had he been more thorough the first time, this physician would have been alerted to a sensorineural hearing loss associated with rubella, and a diagnosis would have been made early. The child would have been fitted with a hearing aid at about the age of one, and would have been enrolled in a program for the hearing handicapped at an earlier time.

The prognosis for this child is not good because accurate diagnosis and treatment were so late. Had a complete medical history been taken, habilitation of this child would have been appropriate and her chances of normal learning and social development would have been maximized.

THE PARENT QUESTIONNAIRE

To facilitate taking an extensive profile in a busy practice, it is recommended that the physician ask the child's parents to complete a Parent Questionnaire (see Appendix A at the end of this chapter). Since filling out a questionnaire requires a considerable amount of time, the parents should be asked to complete the questionnaire at home and subsequently to meet with the physician to discuss it.

The Parent Questionnaire represents a composite history, parts of which have been gathered from the following chapters of this text. For instance, the extended family history is designed to help the physician rule out genetic factors. The prenatal, perinatal, and neonatal history helps rule out congenital abnormalities and suspicions of neglect and abuse, as well as neurological disorders; and the developmental history and systemic review assist in the identification of vision, hearing, neuromotor, and speech and language problems.

The first page of the Parent Questionnaire contains an introductory paragraph to the parents. It is important for the physician to explain why their participation is necessary when giving the questionnaire to the parents. The physician can tell them that development is influenced by a large number of factors which all interact, and that he or she is asking them to complete this comprehensive questionnaire so that the development of their child can be fully understood. The physician can explain that the parents are being asked to complete the questionnaire at home so that they can discuss the answers, look up some information in baby and health records, and—when necessary—consult previous physicians and other professionals who have cared for the child.

Because the parents are asked to return the questionnaire to the physician prior to meeting with him or her, the physician has time to review the answers and identify sections that require further explanation. Thus, it is possible to review the history with the parents in a minimum amount of time.

The questionnaire is divided into the following usual categories:

1. background information pertaining to the family;
2. initial information regarding the history of the present illness;
3. pregnancy history as it relates to the present illness;
4. birth history;
5. health or past medical history, including the systemic review;
6. developmental history;
7. school or educational history;
8. activities of daily living;
9. dental history;
10. family history;
11. pregnancy history of the mother;
12. environmental history.

The final page asks the parents to list the names and addresses of professionals who have had previous contact with the child. Also provided is a sample Release of Information form that parents are requested to complete for each professional and facility listed (see Appendix B). It is important that the parents be provided with sufficient Release of Information forms so that they can complete one for each relevant professional and facility that is listed.

Physicians who have not previously utilized such a questionnaire expect that parents will not complete it. That fortunately turns out not to be the case; virtually all parents, even those who have not been privileged to have much education, do complete all or most of the questionnaire. Indeed, most parents seem pleased when the physician requests that they fill out the history questionnaire. A common complaint from parents is that physicians don't sit down and spend time with them; they see the history-taking approach as proof that their physician really does care, and that he or she also has skills beyond those they have experienced in the past.

For a further elaboration on the use of the Parent Questionnaire in evaluating the child's home environment, a reference work accompanies this chapter. It is entitled *Environmental Evaluation,* and is written by Dr. Henry L. Fischer, a psychologist with an extensive private practice which deals with developmentally delayed children (see Supplemental Reading).

THE PARENT INTERVIEW

In arranging the parent interview, it is helpful to schedule an hour's time during which both the physician and the parents can give undivided attention to a discussion of the child's history. Since the child would be a distraction during such a session, the parents should not bring the child to this meeting. Similarly, the physician must set aside an appropriate amount of time free from interruptions. Some physicians reserve a particular time of the week for parent interviews. Scheduling of the interview and the sequence of topics for discussion will be determined by the physician's preference and office procedure; however, it is important that sufficient time be allotted so that all aspects of the questionnaire can be covered and additional information can be gained from the parents' responses.

To assist in the recording of complete information about the child's current condition, the History of the Present Illness form (Appendix C) includes key words as reminders of important points to consider. These reminders should enable the physician to obtain a complete picture of the nature of the child's present condition and of the occurrences which prompted the parents to seek medical assistance.

Depending upon the nature of the problem, the age of the child, and the parents' ability to narrate the history, a parent interview generally does not take more than an hour. Certainly it can be taken in less time. But since the developmental status of the child is governed by a complex interaction of biological (sensory, neurological, genetic, metabolic, etc.) and environmental factors, it is essential that each factor that may be the cause of the developmental delay be ruled out. Even though the physician may believe he or she knows the major cause of a delay—such as a metabolic disorder—without taking a complete history, the physician cannot be certain of the extent to which other factors may also have deterred the child's development.

THE MEDICAL EXAMINATION

Upon completion of the parent interview, it is necessary to schedule an appointment to examine the child. To facilitate the examination of a child who is able to comprehend an explanation of it, it is helpful to have the parents prepare the child beforehand. This preparation consists of having the parent tell the child that the physician will play some games with him or her, such as peeking through a hole to identify pictures, looking at picture books, putting on earphones like a spaceman, and checking how the child can run, skip, jump, and balance on one leg. Depending upon whether or not the child is anxious about the examination, the parents can also act this out with him or her. Such preparation often pays handsome dividends in promoting the child's cooperation, which in turn is reflected in a more accurate assessment in less time with less anxiety to the child.

The Medical Examination form, like the history, represents a combination of a typical pediatric evaluation with selected additions to identify conditions that may cause the child to be delayed in development. It has been included as Appendix D.

Many of the examination items have been taken from subsequent lessons in this training program. For instance, the "Mother-Child Relationship" section is designed to help identify psychological disorders, and the "bruises, scars, and burns" notation under the heading labeled "Skin" is to remind the physician to check for signs of child abuse and/or neglect. The items preceded with an asterisk are to assist the physician in recalling some of the more common congenital abnormalities; the items marked with an "N" are of possible neurological significance.

SUMMARY

This chapter has first discussed a printed medical-developmental questionnaire which the physician should give to the parents of a suspect child to take home and complete. To assure that the parents are motivated to complete the questionnaire, the physician should explain that a child's development is influenced by many interacting factors, each of which must be considered in evaluating their child. By taking the questionnaire home, parents can reflect upon the answers, and in some cases can consult records which they may have kept.

The second point of this lesson was that upon receipt and review of the history questionnaire, the physician should set up an appointment to meet with the parents, without the child present. With the parents, the physician should review the questionnaire and take a history of the present illness.

Upon completion of the history, the physician should schedule the parents to bring the child to the office for a physical examination and other evaluations.*

---

*Printed Parent Questionnaires, along with History and Medical Examination forms and the major checklists in this text may be ordered from: LADOCA Publishing Foundation, East 51st Avenue at Lincoln Street, Denver, Colorado 80216 (telephone 303-629-6379).

APPENDIX A

Parent Questionnaire

This questionnaire concerns you and your child. Following the referral of your child to us, we are asking you to complete this questionnaire to assist us in focusing on the questions and concerns which you have, and to better understand your child. Some of the information requested may not seem related to your child or his/her problems, but often such seemingly unrelated information becomes very important in our understanding your questions. You may not immediately remember the answers to all of the questions; additional information can often be found by looking through baby books, calling your physician, or talking to relatives. Please try to answer as many of the questions as possible. *If there is not enough space to answer a question, please use the back of the sheet.*

If you do not understand any of the questions, call us at _____
and ask to speak to_____, who will assist you.

GENERAL INFORMATION

Date_____

Child's Name_____Birthdate_____Age_____Sex: M F

Home Address_____Phone_____

_____
County   City   State   Zip Code

Natural Father_____Birthdate_____

  Occupation_____Religion_____

  Ethnic Background_____Years of Schooling_____

  Health_____

Natural Mother_____Birthdate_____

  Occupation_____Religion_____

  Ethnic Background_____Years of Schooling_____

  Health_____

Who referred you here for evaluation?_____

[N]What is it about your child which concerns you?_____

_____

_____

_____

[N]When was it first noticed?_____

What have you been told with regard to the problem?_____

_____

_____

_____

What things do you presently *not* understand about your child?_____

_____

_____

_____

[N]Of possible neurological significance

How do you think that we might be able to help you?_____

_____

_____

_____

How do you feel your child can best be helped?_____

_____

_____

_____

<u>PREGNANCY</u>

Questions in this and the following section refer to the pregnancy of the child whose problem has caused you to seek assistance.

Did you have any problems getting pregnant?_____

Was this a planned pregnancy?_____Feelings about being pregnant_____

_____

During which month did you start prenatal care?_____Where?_____

Weight before pregnancy_____Weight gain_____

[N]Any weight loss in any part of pregnancy?_____If so, when?_____

[N]Medicines taken and when (include all medications, such as vitamins, birth control pills, etc., including aspirin if taken frequently)_____

_____

Did you smoke during the pregnancy?_____If so, when?_____

How many cigarettes per day?_____

[N]How much alcohol did you consume during your pregnancy?_____

Number of alcoholic drinks per week_____If so, when?_____

[N]Any narcotic drugs during or prior to this pregnancy?_____

[N]Any illnesses?____If so, when?_____

[N]Did you have any fever during pregnancy? 1st 3 mo.___ 2nd 3 mo.___ last 3 mo._____

If so, how high was fever?_____For how long did it persist?_____hours or_____days

[N]X-rays during or shortly before pregnancy?_____[N]Vaginal bleeding?_____

[N]High blood pressure?_____Much morning sickness?_____Much swelling?_____

[N]Hospitalizations?_____

^NOperations?_____

^NAccidents?_____

Unusual worries?_____

Special diet?_____

^NWhen did you first feel the baby move?_____

How were the baby's movements during pregnancy?

    _____Stronger than expected
    _____Weaker than expected
    _____About the same as expected

BIRTH HISTORY

^NWas the baby born on time, early, or late?_____

^NWas any stimulation of labor used?_____Type_____

^NLength of labor in hours_____Length of hard labor_____

Length of time before delivery that bag of waters broke_____

^NType of anesthesia or pain relief:

    Sedative_____   Shot for pain relief_____

    Spinal or caudal_____   Gas or Pentothal_____

Were you awake when the baby was born?_____

^NType of delivery:

    Natural (vaginal)_____   Breech_____

    Cesarean section_____   Forceps_____

Mother's blood group (ABO)_____   Mother's Rh factor_____

Baby's blood group (ABO)_____   Baby's Rh factor_____

^NBaby's birth weight_____Birth length_____Head circumference_____

^NInfant's condition:

    Breathed immediately_____   Cried immediately_____

    Required oxygen_____   Length of stay in nursery_____

    Seizures or fits_____

Problems during the first week (i.e., incubator, yellow skin, feeding difficulties, bleeding tendency, infection, etc.):_____

Medicines given during hospital stay_____

Later hospitalizations of child:

    Name of Hospital   *Date*   *Reason*

_____

_____

_____

_____

_____

_____

HEALTH

Breast or bottle fed_____ [N]Did child eat well?_____

[N]Sleep patterns_____

[N]Childhood diseases (list age and anything unusual about any of them):

    Mumps_____   3-day (or German) measles_____

    Chicken pox_____   7-day (or red) measles_____

    Roseola_____   Scarlet fever_____

    Whooping cough_____   Serious illness_____

Immunizations (dates or ages received and any unusual reactions):

    DPT series_____   Smallpox_____

    DPT booster_____   Measles_____

    Polio (oral)_____   Mumps_____

If your child has had any of the following, please indicate and explain details:

[N]Accidents_____

[N]High fever, unknown cause_____

Pneumonia_____

Anemia_____

[N]Urine infection or disease_____

[N]Problem in bladder or bowel control_____

[N]Constipation_____

[N]Does your child have trouble seeing?_____

[N]Do your child's eyes turn in or out, or are they ever not straight?_____

[N]Crossed eyes_____

[N]Speech problems_____

[N]Difficulty eating or feeding self_____

[N]Difficulties in: Swallowing_____Chewing_____Drooling_____

[N]Hearing problems_____

[N]Frequent ear infections_____

[N]Foot problems (any special shoes, braces, etc.)_____

[N]Skin disease or abnormality_____

Allergies_____

[N]Birthmarks_____

[N]Seizures or convulsions_____

Unusual fears_____

[N]Sleeping difficulties and night terrors_____

[N]Head banging_____

[N]Rocking_____

[N]Breath holding_____

Temper tantrums_____

Discipline problem_____

[N]Ingestion of drugs, cleaners, or non-food items_____

Other illnesses_____

_____

DEVELOPMENT

We would like to have information about some of the developmental milestones of your child. Indicate the age in months when your child first did each of the following. (Indicate that the child has not yet done it by writing "No;" if you do not remember write "NR.") Please be as specific as possible in pinpointing the age.

[N]Held head erect_____   [N]Sat alone_____

[N]Rolled over front to back_____   [N]Crawled_____

N Rolled over back to front_____   N Pulled to stand_____

N Stood alone_____   N Smiled spontaneously_____

N Walked holding on furniture_____   N Fed self cookie_____

N Walked without holding_____   N Drank from cup_____

N Ran with good control_____   N Played pat-a-cake, peek-a-boo, or
                                                      bye-bye_____
N Walked up steps_____
                                                    N Recognized parents_____
N Rode tricycle_____
                                                    N Showed fear with strangers_____
N Said "ma-ma" or "da-da"_____
                                                    N Used spoon without spilling much_____
N Used word (other than "ma-ma" or "da-da")
  with meaning_____   N Toilet training started_____

N Repeated sounds others made_____   N Toilet training finished_____

N Said three single words_____   N Put on clothes_____

N Combined different words_____   N Used sentences_____

N Repeated words others said_____

N Is your child left- or right-handed?_____

N When did you first notice a hand preference?_____

SCHOOLS

Has child ever been in preschool?_____When and where?_____

_____

List schools that child has attended:

   Name of School   *Dates*

_____

_____

_____

_____

_____

N Has your child ever been held back in school?_____

_____

[N]Has child ever been in special education? If so, when, where, and what kind?

_____

[N]Has child ever been in remedial classes? If so, when, where, and what kind?

_____

[N]Has child ever had special tutoring? If so, when, where, and by whom?_____

_____

[N]Has child ever received speech therapy? If so, when, where, and by whom?_____

_____

[N]Has child ever received any other type of therapy? If so, please describe_____

_____

Describe any school problems that you are presently aware of_____

_____

_____

_____

ACTIVITIES

[N]What things does your child like to do?_____

_____

_____

[N]What things does your child do well?_____

_____

_____

[N]What things present the greatest difficulty for your child?_____

_____

_____

[N]Describe play indoors_____

_____

_____

[N]Describe play outdoors_____

_____

_____

[N]How does your child play and/or get along with other children?_____

_____

_____

Give detailed description of an average day_____

_____

_____

_____

_____

_____

_____

_____

_____

DENTAL HISTORY

Has your child ever been examined by a dentist?_____

For what reason?_____

When was your child's last visit to the dentist?_____

Name and office address of your child's dentist_____

_____

_____

FAMILY HISTORY

Please indicate whether there are any relatives of the child (including parents, grand-parents, aunts, uncles, and cousins), who have the same or a similar problem for which you are seeking evalution. Also indicate for these persons whether there are serious, chronic, or recurrent illnesses or abnormalities such as [N]*birth defects*, [N]*miscarriages*, [N]*diabetes*, [N]*convulsions* or *epilepsy (fits)*, mental or emotional disorders, slow development, mental retardation, school problems, [N]*cerebral palsy*, [N]*muscular disorders*, cancers, leukemia, [N]*thyroid disease (goiter)*, [N]*deafness* or *blindness*, [N]*speech* or *language problems*, [N]*reading* or *learning disorders*. (Please be as specific as possible, giving relationship to child, age of relative and problem.)

Mother_____

Mother's mother_____

Mother's father_____

Mother's brothers and sisters_____

Mother's maternal grandmother_____

Mother's maternal grandfather_____

Mother's paternal grandmother_____

Mother's paternal grandfather_____

Mother's aunts and uncles_____

Mother's cousins_____

Father_____

Father's mother_____

Father's father_____

Father's brothers and sisters_____

Father's maternal grandmother_____

Father's maternal grandfather_____

Father's paternal grandmother_____

Father's paternal grandfather_____

Father's aunts and uncles_____

Father's cousins_____

Describe any family tensions_____

List support sources outside the family (relatives, friends)_____

_____

Future goals of child's father_____

_____

Future goals of child's mother_____

_____

PREGNANCY HISTORY

Past pregnancies of child's mother: Number of times pregnant_____

Longest period of infertility_____

NLive births_____ NStillbirths_____ NMiscarriages_____

List dates of past pregnancies. Indicate if there was: a miscarriage; threatened miscarriage (bleeding); premature birth; twins; deformity or other difficulty with live-born children; or any other complications. Please list any birth defects, however unimportant you consider them.

Name	Birthdate	Birth Weight	Grade in School	Any School or Health Problems

N Are the mother and father cousins, or in any other way related?_____

Previous marriage of either parent? If so, to whom, date, and date of divorce_____

Please list children of either parent born prior to this marriage:

Name	Birthdate	Birth Weight	Grade in School	Any School or Health Problems

<u>ENVIRONMENT</u>

Who lives in home besides child, parents, brothers, and sisters? List age, relation, and health:

_____

List members of the family not living at home, where living, and reason:_____

_____

Has your child ever been separated from the family? If so, list age, duration, and reason:

_____

Any recent major family problem such as death, illness, separation, or accident?_____

_____

Do you speak more than one language at home?_____

Date of marriage of child's parents_____

If appropriate, date of separation_____Date of divorce_____

Step- or adopted father_____   Birthdate_____

    Occupation_____   Religion_____

    Ethnic background_____   Years of schooling_____

    Health_____

Step- or adopted mother_____   Birthdate_____

    Occupation_____   Religion_____

    Ethnic background_____   Years of schooling_____

    Health_____

_____

                Signature of Reviewer

In order to have a better understanding of your child's particular needs, it is important to gather background information from some of the following places and persons. Please list their names and addresses and complete and sign a Release of Information form for each.

	Name	*Address*	*City*	*State*
Doctor who delivered child:				
Hospital where child was born:				
Places where child has received care: Hospitals or agencies (welfare, visiting nurse service, speech, occupational or physical therapy, psychiatrist, etc.)				
Physicians who have cared for your child:				
Schools child has attended:				

Signature_____

Relationship_____

Date_____

APPENDIX B

Release of Information

Date:_____

To:_____

Please give information from your case records of:

_____

_____

Birthdate:_____

Signed:_____

Relationship:_____

Witness:_____

One form should be completed for each person or agency from whom information is being requested.

After parents have completed this form, they should return it with the Parent Questionnaire to their child's physician.

APPENDIX C

History of the Present Illness

Name _____ Date _____

Nature of Problem(s)
Parent Perception of Function

^NDevelopmental Problem(s)
    Onset
    Course

^NEpisodic Events
    Seizures
    Fainting

^NExposures

Related Factors

Previous Evaluation(s)

Previous Treatment

Explore Significant Answers
    from Parent Questionnaire

^NPrecipitating Events
    Pregnancy
    Birth

Neonatal
Trauma
Congenital heart disease
Meningitis
Encephalitis
Seizures
Other illnesses

Family History
    For same problem
    Other problem(s)
    Miscarriages
    Infant deaths
    Birth deaths
    Consanguinity

Developmental History
    Gross motor
    Fine motor-adaptive
    Language
    Personal/social

_____
Signature of Person Taking
The History

[N] Of possible neurological significance

APPENDIX D

Medical Examination

Name _____ Date _____

^{N}Weight ____, ____%; Height ____, ____%; OFC ____, ____%; P ____; R ____; BP ____

GENERAL OBSERVATION

Mother-Child Relationship:
    Body contact, visual and verbal interaction, mother's sensitivity to child's needs
    Reaction to separation from mother
    Older child: memories and dreams

^{N}*General Activity:*
    Type and amount
    Stereotypic behavior

^{N}*Speech and Language:*
    How does child listen
    Comprehension of language
    How does child talk
    If not talking, how communicate
    Difference in communication between child and family and child and examiner

Appearance:
    Stature, body build
    Posture
    Unusual odors
    Nutritional status
    Cleanliness

EXAMINATION

^{N}*Skin:*
    Texture, hyper- and hypopigmentation
    Birthmarks (note size and location)
    Bruises, scars, burns

Head:
    ^{N}Shape, sutures
    Facies
    *Hair (texture, whorls)
    *Hairline
    ^{N}Fontanelle(s)

Eyes:
    *Slant
    *Spacing
    *Epicanthal folds
    *Brushfield spots
    *Palpebral fissures
    ^{N}Strabismus (pupilary light reflex test)
            (alternate cover test)

    ^{N}Cornea
    ^{N}Sclera, conjunctiva
    ^{N}Pupils (equality)
    ^{N}Iris
    ^{N}Lens
    ^{N}Retina (disc and vessels)
    ^{N}Macula

^{N}*Ears:*
    *Placement
    *Pinna
    *Tags
    *Canals
    TMs
    Sinus tracts

Nose:
    *Nasal bridge
    *Shape
    Other

Mouth:
    *Size, shape
    ^{N}Tongue
    ^{N}*Palate
    Teeth
    ^{N}Pharynx
    Jaw

Neck:
    *Length
    *Skinfolds
    Masses
    Other

Chest and Back:
    *Shape
    *Scoliosis
    *Nipples, breasts
    ^{N}Heart
    Lung fields

Abdomen:
    *Umbilical hernia
    ^{N}Organomegaly
    Other

Genital and Anal Areas:
    Hygiene
    N Echymosis, hematomas, lacterations
    Vulvar vestibule (discharge, increased
        size of vaginal opening, hymen
        intactness)
    Anus intactness

Extremities:
    N Range of motion
    N* Symmetry

N* Proportion of body
N* Finger, hand size and shape
 *Clinodactyly, syndactyly
 *Nails
 *Palmar creases
  Toes and thumbs

_____

Signature of Examiner

*Minor anomalies
N Of possible neurological significance

SUPPLEMENTAL READING:
ENVIRONMENTAL EVALUATION

Henry L. Fischer, Ph.D.

IMPORTANCE OF ENVIRONMENTAL EVALUATION

The primary care physician is in a unique position to evaluate handicapped children and their families. Thus the physician plays a very important role in exploring the environmental context and social-emotional qualities of those families. Knowledge of the family's emotional environment will help determine: how readily the handicapped child will be accepted into the family community; how successful the child's development of self-esteem will be; how successful or unsuccessful any future treatment programs will be for the child; and the ultimate achievement level of the child.

One use of an environmental assessment is in determining the extent to which a child's developmental problem may be secondary to a suboptimal home environment. Even when the major causative factor for retardation is known, as in the case of such biological causes as Down Syndrome, phenylketonuria, and prematurity, it is still essential to determine whether the home environment is conductive to optimal development. If suboptimal environmental circumstances are detected, attempts must be made to rectify or supplement this shortcoming so that the child can develop to the limits of his or her capacity.

PRENATAL HISTORY

It is always important for the physician to inquire whether or not there were unsuccessful pregnancies prior to the one which resulted in the handicapped child. The mother may reveal a number of previous pregnancies, the possibility of spontaneous or planned abortions, or the occurrence of a stillbirth. The feelings and stresses associated with these experiences are important to explore. If a physician discovers that there had been a long period before the wife became pregnant, and there were issues of infertility or carefully planned delay of pregnancy, then the physician can question whether there also was some inordinate pressure on the parents to have a child at a certain point in time. The general parental anticipation of having a healthy, normal child is abruptly dashed at the discovery of a child's handicap, and thus it is important for the physician to discover the parents' reaction and ability to cope with this stress.

Naturally, the physician should examine the question of whether the pregnancy which resulted in a handicapped child was a planned or desired pregnancy, whether the pregnancy occurred within or outside of marriage, and whether both husband and wife felt similarly enthusiastic or disappointed about the pregnancy. If the pregnancy was unwanted or illegitimate, it is possible that the parents may look on the handicapped child as a punishment for their real or imagined transgressions. The existence of a genetic defect may be seen similarly as a result of parental "badness," or may be blamed by one parent on the other.

Finally, the general mood of both parents during the pregnancy might have had very important bearing on their ability to be capable parents when the child was born. Often, the occurrence of physical illness, the absence of the father, or important losses or separations during pregnancy can have important bearing on the pregnant woman's mood; these experiences can color her outlook or readiness to be a warm, nurturing parent.

NATAL HISTORY

In taking a natal history, the physician should inquire whether the birth was normal, complicated or premature. Because it is important for the physician to know whether the mother felt strong support from her spouse at birth, the father's absence or presence at that time should be explored. In the event of a complicated birth, it would be important to note whether a child's handicapping condition was related to these complications, or whether the mother in any way felt responsible for them. Frequently, parents express anger or animosity toward professionals who they feel might have been responsible for the complication of the birth. Such feelings might carry over into further relationships with professionals who will later evaluate and attempt to treat the handicapped child. It is also important for the physician to know whether the parents were aware of any difficulties with the child at the time of birth, and whether there was any need for separation due to problems in either mother or child at the time of birth.

INFANCY HISTORY

The very simple and straightforward question, "What kind of a baby was he(she)?" is important for the physician to ask in exploring the infancy period. Often parents will request clarification of this question, but usually it is important to ask them to respond with their first impressions. Parents' first reactions may be that the child was a "good baby," or "fussy." They may respond that the child "cried all the time" or "slept all the time." These answers may give the physician valuable information about parental response to their child from early infancy.

After hearing these first impressions, the physician then should explore the feelings the parents had in caring for a difficult child. The handicapped child who is a fussy eater may be particularly devastating to its mother, since she may feel the child is rejecting her best nurturing efforts. The physician may see that the parents have had strong emotions under the pressure of a handicapped child; he or she may recognize that one parent felt unsupported by the other under difficult circumstances. The physician may also realize that the parents felt very alone and unsupported by friends or relatives. All these are important issues for the physician to pursue when taking a history.

Illnesses, hospitalizations, or separation of either parent from the child should be examined carefully because of their usual strong bearing on later child development. Prolonged hospitalization of the child near the time of birth, for example, can be detrimental to the child's development of appropriate trust and attachment to parents.

With the handicapped child who has experienced frequent illness in early infancy, it is important to ask parents about their relationship to the physicians or other professionals with whom they were dealing at the time. Frequently, parents who are talking to one physician will be reluctant to admit that they were angry or upset with another physician. However, the parents may develop renewed trust and confidence in another doctor if they are allowed to express their anger or frustration. Permitting and encouraging the expression of such feelings may also prevent future "shopping" behavior on the part of these parents.

Parental self-esteem becomes very critical when a child's handicap or difficulty with any of the important developmental tasks begins to reflect on the parents' assessment of themselves. If a mother and father begin their parenting experience feeling inadequate, it is highly unlikely that they will feel any more confident as developmental tasks and requirements become more difficult for the handicapped child.

EARLY CHILDHOOD HISTORY

During a traditional medical history, exploring the developmental landmarks of the child's life between six months and three years of age is routine. For the handicapped child, such a history is especially important. Some overall judgment can be made by the physician as to the accuracy of parental reporting and the investment the parents have had in observing the child's developmental progress. If a parent is overly vague, the physician might wonder whether some other preoccupation affected the parent during the early development; this could result in the parent's inability to focus on and remember the steps of development. If such is the case, then the physician can explore whether there were such extenuating circumstances as the family moving, the mother becoming immediately pregnant again, the beginning recognition of a child's handicap, or some other personal loss such as a relative's or a friend's death. When the physician discovers that a parent has very vague or unusual recollections about the child's development, he or she might question more broadly what the parents' general notions are about development. Naturally, the number and ages of other children in the family are factors that might contribute to vague recollections about the handicapped child.

Consider the example of the mother who begins toilet training at a very early age, i.e. at seven or eight months, because that was the way she experienced toilet training in her own childhood. Such a mother might also feel that early training will free her from the drudgery of diapers, regardless of the child's negative reactions to being pushed into a developmental task for which he or she is not ready. Toilet training and the other accomplishments of the second year which create greater autonomy in the child can cause widely varying reactions in the parent as well. Where toilet training emerges in the history as an area of concern and conflict for the parent, the physician should explore the quality of the conflict. For example, some parents passively allow their child to be completely free about toilet training without any guidelines or supports; others use shame and embarrassment to coerce the child into toilet training. The physician should also determine the pattern of the child's training by asking if whether after toileting was completed, wetting and soiling were reinitiated, or whether toileting has never been totally completed.

PRESCHOOL HISTORY

Between the ages of about three to six years, the issue of the child's ability to separate is important, particularly as it applies to the first formal school experiences. In asking questions about this issue, the physician should try to ascertain whether the problem of separation was greater for the parent or for the child. For parents of a handicapped child, this age period may also be the time when the handicapping condition may have begun to assert itself more clearly. There may be a significant emotional impact when parents see other children of the same age as their child leaving home to go to preschool and kindergarten while their own child may be seen as incapable of these experiences. If the child has been placed in some kind of preschool environment, then the parents can be asked about comments and observations they have received from teachers. This will usually reveal how the child has been doing in a preschool setting. It may also give the physician some insights into the parents' intentions and aspirations for their child as the child begins to confront the handicapping condition in the "real world." Direct phone contact with the child's teacher can give the physician a first-hand perspective on how the child is doing in school.

If, however, a preschool-age handicapped child is not in any kind of school situation, the physician should explore why this is so. Since there is now much greater availability of early childhood stimulation programs for even severely handicapped children, the parent who has not sought out or is not aware of such resources should certainly be given this information.

GENERAL FAMILY INFORMATION

In the course of taking medical and developmental histories, the physician should ask questions about some additional areas of relevance. These are as follows.

1. Knowledge about the size of the family can be helpful in assessing how the handicapped child's special problems will fit into the family community.
2. The birth order of the handicapped child will greatly determine how ready or unprepared parents feel to deal with special problems.

3. Major illnesses and/or difficulties that exist in any of the children or in the parents themselves will possibly cause greater concern among parents of a handicapped child. For example, if one parent is an alcoholic, or if another sibling has a learning disability, these facts may have important implications for the future development of a handicapped child. Unfortunately, such conditions will affect the amount of time and energy parents are able to invest in the handicapped child.
4. The general level of income and the family's socioeconomic status will determine to some extent the reality of what treatment will be available to the developmentally delayed child.
5. If one or both parents are working, the presence of a handicapped child may create greater or lesser stress.
6. The general stability of the marital relationship may affect the handicapped child's development. Often marital tensions can be observed simply in the general interaction between the parents, and frequently it can be seen in the way each parent describes techniques of managing the handicapped child's behavior. It may also emerge in discussion of how the handicapped child has created major changes and shifts in the parents' individual life styles.
7. The academic level, interests, and aspirations of each parent are relevant, as is information about whether either parent ever had difficulties with learning. This becomes particularly critical when learning difficulties exist and special schooling is indicated for the child under evaluation.
8. The physician should determine whether the family has available such supportive people as friends, grandparents, or neighbors. If so, it is important for the physician to know whether the family is willing to use these resources. If the parents refuse such support, physicians should be concerned that they may be punishing themselves unnecessarily. Such refusal may indicate that the parents feel guilty about having a handicapped child, and may feel also that they need to carry all of the responsibility for the child's care as some sort of atonement.
9. One additional major social-emotional issue which the physician should explore is the general direction of the family's goals. These might be in the areas of employment, education, or economic mobility. A physician who is aware of the family's goals for the future will be better able to increase the parents' ability and willingness to accept

recommendations as the evaluation progresses to its conclusion

The physician should end medical and developmental history-taking by allowing some brief period of time for parents to respond to an open-ended question about whether anything has been left out. Frequently, when given the opportunity, parents will raise an issue that has important implications for the social-emotional climate within which the child will grow. Also, they may raise a forgotten point which may have great importance because of the fact that they neglected to mention it until the very end.

SUMMARY

This lesson has addressed itself to how a child's primary care physician, when taking the history and examining the child, can gain a better understanding of the environment in which the child has lived—for the environment promotes or hinders the development of all children. A second reason for such an understanding is to facilitate effective counseling of the parents regarding their child's developmental status, and to make the most effective recommendations for the future. And finally, through an environmental evaluation, the physician can become aware of the parents' life style and aspirations for the future. Only with this information completed can the physician present recommendations for future treatment in the most appropriate manner.

BIBLIOGRAPHY

Anthony, E. J., and Benedek, T. (Eds.). *Parenthood: Its psychology and psychopathology*. Boston: Little, Brown, and Co., 1970.

Fraiberg, S. *The magic years*. New York: Charles Scribner and Sons, 1959.

Mussen, P. H., Conger, J. J., and Kagan, J. *Child development and personality* (4th ed.). New York: Harper and Row, 1974.

Steinhauer, P. D., and Rae-Grant, Q. (Eds.). *Psychological problems of the child and his family*. Toronto: MacMillan of Canada, 1977.

Talbot, N. B., Kagan, J., and Eisenberg, L. *Behavioral science in pediatric medicine*. Philadelphia: W. B. Saunders Company, 1971.

Chapter 5

Goal   To develop skills in the ophthalmological assessment of children suspected of developmental delays, and in appropriate referral to an ophthalmologist.

Objectives   At the end of this chapter, the physician should be able to:
- screen a child for visual acuity;
- demonstrate tests for strabismus;
- recognize significant intraocular abnormalities;
- refer appropriately to an ophthalmologist for evaluation and testing.

OPHTHALMOLOGICAL EVALUATION

By
JAMES SPRAGUE, M.D.

I. Introduction
   A. Ophthalmological problems occur with increased frequency among developmentally delayed children.
   B. Undetected vision abnormalities can add to a handicapped child's developmental problems.
   C. In addition, an ophthalmologic evaluation may give clues to the cause of a delay.
II. Development of Vision
   A. Good vision requires a normal eyeball and central nervous system connections, a sharp optical image, and an intact fixation reflex.
   B. The fixation reflex, which is normally present at about six weeks of age, requires active stimulation up to six or nine years.
   C. A three-year-old should see about 20/50, a four-year-old about 20/40, a five-year-old about 20/30, and a six-year-old about 20/20.
III. Amblyopia
   A. Amblyopia is poor vision in one eye without ophthalmoscopic abnormalities.
   B. The two most common causes of amblyopia are: marked unequal refractive errors in the two eyes; and strabismus, which leads to suppression of the deviated eye.
   C. The presence of amblyopia in children is between three-and-one-half and five percent; the prevalence is higher among children with mental retardation.
   D. Amblyopia can be reversed with optical correction and patching of the good eye if treatment is begun early.
IV. Screening of Visual Acuity
   A. A history of visual problems is often not very helpful in infants, but may be more accurate in older children.
   B. The illiterate "E" test, given to children three years of age and older, is the most accurate.
   C. The picture card test, given to children under three years and older children who are untestable on the "E," requires a verbal response.
   D. The fixation test, which is used for children from three months to two years of age and for older children untestable on the "E" or picture card test, is a gross visual test.
V. Screening for Strabismus
   A. Strabismus occurs with increased frequency in handicapped children; early treatment is most effective.
   B. Strabismus may be a possible warning sign of an intraocular lesion.
   C. Because the history is usually helpful in identifying strabismus in children, the parents should be questioned.
      1. Esotropia is more common than exotropia.

      2. However, intermittent exotropia is more common than intermittent esotropia.

  D. The alternate cover test picks up small deviations, but requires that the test administrator be very close to the child.

  E. The pupillary light reflex test, which is simple to perform and does not require touching the child, may miss small errors.

VI. Rating the Total Test

  A. The total eye test is considered abnormal if the child scored abnormal on any of the three vision tests in either eye, if the child squinted with either eye during testing, or if the history or the pupillary light reflex or alternate cover tests were abnormal.

  B. The total eye test is untestable if the examiner could not test the child's visual acuity or could not be sure the eyes were straight.

  C. If the total test rating was abnormal or untestable, the child should be screened again in a few weeks.

  D. If the child is again untestable or abnormal on rescreening, the child should be referred to an ophthalmologist.

VII. Examination of Intraocular Structures

  A. The cornea can be examined for opacities with a penlight or a direct ophthalmoscope set on the plus (or black) numbers.

  B. The normal cornea is 10 millimeters in diameter at birth, enlarging to the adult size of 12 millimeters during the second six months of life.

  C. Blood in the shallow anterior chamber is a hyphema and indicates a serious ocular injury.

  D. In an infant, the iris appears flat and without the normal stromal clefts.

  E. The dilator fibers of the iris are not fully formed until three or four years of age, making it difficult to check the infant's pupils for constriction on accommodation.

VIII. Dilation

  A. Children with strabismus, poor vision, or a systemic disease should be referred for a dilated fundus examination to an ophthalmologist.

  B. A combination of cyclopentolate and neosynephrine can be used to dilate the pupil.

  C. A topical anaesthetic and lid retractors may be necessary to examine the retina.

IX. Referral Criteria

  A. Leukocoria—or white pupil—which maintains the possibility of retinoblastoma is a criterion for immediate referral.

  B. Bilateral congenital cataracts and monocular cataracts also require referral.

  C. Other indications for referral are true strabismus and poor vision.

X. Summary

INTRODUCTION

It is a well-established fact that ophthalmological problems occur with increased frequency among developmentally delayed children.

For example, when 728 children under the age of six were studied at the Child Evaluation Clinic in Louisville, Kentucky, 49 percent of them were found to have eye problems. These included refractive errors, strabismus, syndromes with eye findings, optic nerve disorders, congenital cataracts, and retinal diseases. Twenty-six percent of the children with eye findings had ocular problems which appeared to contribute to their developmental delays. In fact, it has been estimated by the prominent geneticist, Victor McKusick, that 25 percent of known hereditary conditions in childhood have associated ocular findings.

This and other studies indicate that all children suspected of being developmentally delayed should receive an evaluation for possible accompanying vision problems, since undetected vision abnormalities can add to a handicapped child's developmental problems.

In addition, an ophthalmological evaluation is important because it may give clues to the cause of a delay. Some conditions, such as congenital rubella, cytomegalic inclusion disease, or toxoplasmosis lead to a variety of handicaps, including mental retardation and eye pathology. Thus, careful examination of the eyes may help establish a diagnosis.

DEVELOPMENT OF VISION

Good vision requires a normal eyeball and normal central nervous system connections. It also requires a sharp optical image and an intact fixation reflex. The eye is not fully developed at birth; the macula does not appear in its adult form until about four months of age, and myelination of the optic nerve, which starts centrally and proceeds down the optic tract from the geniculate body into the optic nerve, may not be completed by birth. Therefore, the newborn infant is not expected to have normal vision.

A sharp image is formed by the optical system of the eye if there are no marked refractive errors and if there are no opacities in the optical media. This image, which is formed by the lens and the cornea, is placed on the fovea by the fixation reflex. This reflex is normally present at about six weeks of age and requires active stimulation up to six to nine years of age if vision is to develop. If the fixation reflex is not stimulated—for example, if the child has bilateral, congenital cataracts—then it will never be obtained, and the child will develop searching nystagmus.

Normal vision does not reach 20/20 until about the age of six. One way of remembering the development of normal vision is to remember that the three-year-old should see about 20/50; the four-year-old should see about 20/40; and the five-year-old should see about 20/30.

AMBLYOPIA

A common vision problem is amblyopia. An eye may appear to be developing normally; however, if the fixation reflexes are not stimulated equally, a child is at risk of developing amblyopia (poor vision in the eye without ophthalmoscopic abnormalities).

The two most common causes of amblyopia are: first, markedly unequal refractive errors in the two eyes, so that one eye does not get as sharp an image on the retina as the other; and second, strabismus, which leads to suppression of the deviated eye.

The presence of amblyopia in normal children has been estimated to be between three-and-one-half and five percent; the prevalence is higher among children with mental retardation.

Amblyopia can be reversed with optical correction and patching of the good eye to force the child to use the amblyopic eye. This treatment, however, is only effective when the visual-sensory system acts as though it is in a state of flux, which is before the age of six to nine years; it becomes more difficult to correct in the older child. Consequently, amblyopia should be treated early, and therefore, it must be detected early.

SCREENING OF VISUAL ACUITY

In the infant, the history for visual problems is often not very helpful. If the mother reports that the child does not see, she is often correct. The mother may think that the child does see, however, because the child turns to her in feeding, or turns its head in response to tactile or auditory stimuli.

In the older child—toddlers, for example—the parents may have some idea of visual acuity based on how well the child identifies toys, picks things off the floor, or recognizes common roadside signs. How close the child sits to the television set is not a reliable indicator of visual acuity, since most children seem to prefer to sit very close.

The three basic tests for determining visual acuity are the illiterate "E" test for the older preschool child, the picture cards for toddlers, and the fixation test for infants and toddlers. Steps in administering these three tests are listed in Appendix A.

The "E" test is given to children three years of age and older. The "E" is the most accurate of the three tests, but younger children or those who are mentally retarded may not be able to perform it.

The picture card test is given to children under three years of age and to older children who are untestable on the illiterate "E." While not as accurate as the "E," the picture cards are more accurate than the fixation test. A major limitation of the cards is that they require a verbal response, which may be difficult for normal children; retarded children may not recognize the cards, or may be unable to verbalize a response.

The fixation test can be used for children from three months to two years of age, and for children who are unable to do either the illiterate "E" or the picture card test. The advantage of the fixation test is that it doesn't require the child to verbalize or comprehend verbal instructions; the disadvantage is that it is a gross visual test.

SCREENING FOR STRABISMUS

After checking visual acuity, the physician should determine if the child has evidence of strabismus—that is, if the child is cross-eyed or wall-eyed. There is an increased prevalence of strabismus in physically and mentally handicapped children, which has been estimated to be as high as 40 or 50 percent. Amblyopia frequently follows strabismus, and the longer it remains untreated, the more difficult it is to treat.

In addition, strabismus should be thought of as a possible warning sign of an intraocular lesion. For example, 20 percent of children with retinoblastoma, a tumor, first present with strabismus.

Usually the history is helpful in identifying strabismus in children. Although esotropia (eyes that turn in) is more common than exotropia (eyes that turn out), intermittent exotropia is more common than intermittent esotropia. Therefore, if the child's eyes appear straight but the parent describes intermittent exotropia, the physician should reevaluate the child. While the parents may not be able to report which eye turns (indeed, they may not be able to remember whether the eye turns in or out), they probably have noticed that there is something unusual about the way the child's eyes are aligned.

When checking for strabismus, the physician should first ask the parents if they have ever noticed nonstraight eyes. Then the alternate cover test and the pupillary light reflex test should be conducted. Appendix B lists the steps in administering these tests for strabismus.

The alternate cover test picks up small deviations. However, to do this test the administrator must be very close to the child, which is sometimes a disadvantage.

The pupillary light reflex test is simple to perform and can be conducted without touching the child. Its disadvantage is that it may miss small errors.

RATING THE TOTAL TEST

Appendix C, the Eye Tests Scoring Form, provides a method of scoring both the tests for visual acuity and for strabismus.

The total eye test is considered abnormal if:

1. the child was scored abnormal on any of the three vision tests in either eye;
2. the child squinted with either eye during testing; or
3. the history or either the pupillary light reflex or the alternate cover test were abnormal.

The total eye test is considered untestable if:

1. the examiner could not test the child's visual acuity; or
2. the examiner could not be sure that the child's eyes were straight.

If the total test rating was either abnormal or untestable, the child should be screened again in a few weeks. If on rescreening the child is again untestable, he or she should be referred. If the vision screening was abnormal, the child should also be referred—preferably to an ophthalmologist.

EXAMINATION OF INTRAOCULAR STRUCTURES

The third objective in this lesson is to enable the physician to recognize common abnormalities during examination of the eye. Only through looking into the eye can such problems as lens and vitreous opacities, optic nerve anomalies, and retinal anomalies be identified.

In examining the eye, the physician should first examine the cornea for opacities with a penlight or with the direct ophthalmoscope set on the plus (or black) numbers.

Corneal size can be estimated by holding a ruler up to the eye and measuring the diameter of the outer borders of the visible iris. The normal cornea is 10 millimeters in diameter at birth, with the cornea enlarging to the adult size of 12 millimeters during the second six months of life.

The anterior chamber—the space between the cornea and the iris—is shallow in infants. Blood in this space is a hyphema and indicates a serious ocular injury.

In an infant, the iris appears flat and without the normal stromal clefts. The pupils are round and equal in size; they react to light both directly and consensually.

It is frequently difficult to examine pupillary responses in an infant, particularly one with dark irides, because the pupils are so small; this is because the dilator fibers of the iris are not fully formed until three or four years of age. It is difficult to check the infant's pupils for constriction on accommodation. Most Caucasian infants have blue irides, which may not develop their adult color until about two years of age.

DILATION

The busy practitioner often does not have the time to do a dilated fundus examination. Furthermore, the physician will probably refer to an ophthalmologist most of the children whom it would be desirable to dilate. These would include children with strabismus, poor vision, or a systemic disease associated with a high incidence of intraocular problems. However, there may be occasions when it is important for the physician to look inside an eye.

Parasympatholytic or sympathomimetic drugs will dilate the pupil. Cyclomydril® (Alcon Laboratories) is a combination of cyclopentolate, a parasympatholytic, and of neosynephrine, a sympathomimetic. One drop is placed in the eye at intervals of 15 to 30 minutes up to a total of two to four drops, until the pupils dilate.

Once the pupils are dilated, it may still be difficult to examine the retina without using lid retractors. Topical anaesthetic is used to anaesthetize and to wet the cornea. The retractors are placed under the upper and lower lids; an assistant retracts the lids and keeps the cornea moistened with normal saline or artificial tears.

The posterior segment of the eye can then be examined with the direct ophthalmoscope. If the direct ophthalmoscope is set on the plus side (the black numbers), opacities in the lens can be seen in retroillumination. The lens dial is then turned counterclockwise to the minus (or red) numbers, until the retina is in focus.

REFERRAL CRITERIA

There are several intraocular conditions which require immediate referral.

These are as follows.

1. One such condition is leukocoria—or white pupil—which maintains the possibility of retinoblastoma.
2. Bilateral congenital cataracts are also an indication for immediate referral because of the risk of irreversible amblyopia if the fixation reflexes are not stimulated at an early age.
3. Monocular cataracts suggest the possibility of intraocular disease. As an isolated finding, the prognosis for good vision with monocular cataracts is poor because the child prefers the normal eye and the eye on which there has been surgery becomes amblyopic.
4. Strabismus requires referral since it rarely improves spontaneously and since many believe that it responds best to early correction.
5. Poor vision is the final indication for referral for examination and particularly cycloplegic refraction—that is, with parasympatholytic drops. This referral should be to an ophthalmologist.

SUMMARY

This chapter has discussed screening for visual acuity through use of the illiterate "E," the picture cards, and the fixation tests. It has also examined methods of detecting strabismus through questioning parents and through use of the alternate cover and pupillary light reflex tests.

Some common intraocular findings have been discussed, as have indications for dilation and referral.

It is hoped that this chapter has alerted the primary care physician to the increased incidence of poor vision and eye disease among developmentally delayed children. Because untreated vision problems can add to a handicapped child's other problems, and because ophthalmologic evaluation of a suspect child may give clues to the cause of a delay, it is recommended that screening tests and examinations of the eye be conducted on every child suspected of having a developmental delay.

BIBLIOGRAPHY

Edwards, W. C., Price, W. D., and Weisskopf, B. Ocular findings in developmentally handicapped children. *Journal of Pediatric Ophthalmology*, 1972, *9*, 162–167.

Francois, J. Genetic aspects of ophthalmology. *International Ophthalmology Clinics*, 1968, 8 (Whole No. 4).

Goldberg, M. (Ed.). *Genetic and metabolic eye disease*. Boston: Little, Brown and Co., 1974.

Harley, R. D. (Ed.). *Pediatric ophthalmology*. Philadelphia: W. B. Saunders Company, 1975.

Liebman, S. D., and Gellis, S. S. *The pediatrician's ophthalmology*. St. Louis: C. V. Mosby, 1966.

McKusick, V. A. *Mendelian inheritance in man*. Baltimore: Johns Hopkins Press, 1966.

Ophthalmologic Staff of the Hospital for Sick Children. *The eye in childhood*. Toronto: Yearbook Medical Publishers, 1967.

Parks, M. M. *Ocular mobility and strabismus*. New York: Harper and Row, 1975.

Shaefer, W. W., and Weiss, D. I. *Congenital and pediatric glaucomas*. St. Louis: C. V. Mosby, 1970.

Simons, K., and Reinecke, R. D. Amblyopia screening and stereopsis. In *Symposium on strabismus: Transactions of the New Orleans Academy of Ophthalmology*. St. Louis: C. V. Mosby, 1977.

Tasman, R. *Retinal diseases in children*. New York: Harper and Row, 1971.

Van Noorden, G. K. Amblyopia: Basic concepts and current treatment. In *Symposium on strabismus: Transactions of the New Orleans Academy of Ophthalmology*. St. Louis: C. V. Mosby, 1977.

APPENDIX A

*Steps in Administering Tests for Visual Acuity**

Checklist "E" Test

	Correct	Incorrect
1. Demonstrates how "E" points while near child.		
2. Turns the card and asks child to point in direction of the "E".		
3. Demonstrates use of occluder and asks child to peek through hole.		
4. Measures 15 feet.		
5. Shows child large "E" at 15 feet and asks direction pointing.		
6. Shows child smaller "E" and asks direction pointing.		
7. Covers "E" while rotating card.		
8. Tests until 3 correct or 3 incorrect responses given		
9. Adequate lighting used.		
10. Other eye tested.		
11. Results recorded properly on form		
12. Results scored accurately		

Checklist Picture Card Test

	Correct	Incorrect
1. Asks child to name each of 7 pictures (if wrong name or no name given, screener gives correct name or double-checks incorrect name)		
2. Demonstrates use of occluder.		
3. Measures 15 feet.		
4. Shows child picture cards at 15 feet distance		
5. Tests until 3 correct or 3 incorrect responses are given (whichever is first).		
6. Adequate lighting used.		
7. Other eye tested.		
8. Results recorded properly on form		
9. Results scored accurately		

Checklist Fixation Test

	Correct	Incorrect
1. Screener 1½ feet from child		
2. Flashlight held close to examiner's eyes.		
3. One eye of child covered.		
4. Child's attention attracted to light or spinning toy.		
5. Flashlight moved to the right and left.		
6. Other eye tested.		
7. Results recorded properly on form		
8. Results scored accurately		

*From Frankenburg, W. K., Goldstein, A. D., and Barker, J., *Denver Eye Screening Test Manual/Workbook,* University of Colorado Medical Center, 1973.

APPENDIX B

Steps in Administering Tests for Strabismus*

Checklist Cover Test

	Correct	Incorrect
1. Covers one of child's eyes with hand or thumb without touching the face or eyes		
2. Flashlight held near own face		
3. Moves light slightly to attract attention		
4. Moves hand or thumb to cover other eye.		
5. Moves hand or thumb at proper speed		
6. Interprets results correctly.		
7. Scores results correctly.		

Checklist Pupillary Light Reflex Test

	Correct	Incorrect
1. Flashlight held just below examiner's eyes.		
2. Distance 1½ feet from face of child		
3. Position of light reflection in pupils observed		
4. Interprets results correctly.		
5. Scores results correctly.		

*From Frankenburg, W. K., Goldstein, A. D., and Barker, J., *Denver Eye Screening Test Manual/Workbook,* University of Colorado Medical Center, 1973.

APPENDIX C

*Eye Tests Scoring Form**

Name_____Hospital Number_____Ward_____

Address_____

	FIRST SCREENING: DATE						RESCREENING: DATE					
	Right Eye			Left Eye			Right Eye			Left Eye		
Vision Tests	Normal	Abnormal	Untestable	Normal	Abnormal	Untestable	Normal	Abnormal	Untestable	Normal	Abnormal	Untestable
1. "E" (3 years and above; 3 to 5 trials).	3P	3F	U	3P	3F	U	3P	3F	U	3P	3F	U
2. Picture Card (2 1/2 to 2 11/12 years; 3 to 5 trials)	3P	3F	U	3P	3F	U	3P	3F	U	3P	3F	U
3. Fixation (6 months to 2 5/12 years).	P	F	U	P	F	U	P	F	U	P	F	U
4. Squinting		YES			YES			YES			YES	

	Normal	Abnormal	Untestable	Normal	Abnormal	Untestable
Tests for Non-Straight Eyes						
1. Do your child's eyes turn in or out, or are they ever not straight?	NO	YES	U	NO	YES	U
2. Cover Test.	P	F	U	P	F	U
3. Pupillary Light Reflex. . . .	P	F	U	P	F	U

Total Test Rating (Both Eyes)		
Normal (passed vision test plus no squint, plus passed 2/3 tests for non-straight eyes).	Normal	Normal
Abnormal (abnormal on any vision test, squinting, or 2 of 3 procedures for non-straight eyes). .	Abnormal	Abnormal
Untestable (untestable on any vision test or untestable on 2/3 tests for non-straight eyes). . .	Untestable	Untestable
Future Rescreening Appointment for Total Test Rating (Abnormal or Untestable)	Date:	Date:

*From Frankenburg, W. K., Goldstein, A. D., and Barker, J., *Denver Eye Screening Test Manual/Workbook,* Univ. of Colo. Medical Center, 1973.

Chapter 6

Goal   To develop skills in the audiological evaluation of children with developmental delays.

Objectives   At the end of this chapter, the physician should be able to:
- describe two types of hearing loss, their causes, and how they are treated;
- list prenatal, perinatal, postnatal, and preschool-age medical factors which cause auditory acuity impairment in children;
- apply the hearing developmental history to elicit parental concern;
- identify children who need additional hearing assessment procedures;
- refer children appropriately to an audiologist or an otolaryngologist.

AUDIOLOGICAL EVALUATION

By
JERRY NORTHERN, Ph.D.

I. Importance of Hearing Screening
 Hearing impairment affects the child's intellectual and social development.

II. Prevalence of Hearing Loss
 A. Three to four thousand profoundly deaf babies are born in the U.S. annually.
 B. Another 5,000 have significant hearing impairments that require special education or rehabilitation.
 C. As many as 15 percent of preschool children have mild to moderate hearing losses which are medically or surgically remediable.
 D. Prevalence of hearing loss is greater among Eskimos, Navajo Indians, inner city populations, and among children with cleft palate, Down Syndrome and cranio-facial disorders.

III. Significance of Hearing Loss to the Child
 A. Undetected hearing problems can impair a child's intellectual and social development.
 B. Developmental delay and communication problems are often associated with hearing losses.

IV. Conductive and Sensorineural Hearing Losses
 A. Conductive losses involve problems with the sound conduction mechanism.
  1. Conductive losses account for 95 percent of hearing losses among infants and preschool children.
  2. Common causes of this type of loss include: foreign objects in the ear canal, debris in the external auditory canal, external otitis, and problems associated with tympanic membrane mobility.
  3. About 95 percent of all conductive hearing losses can be ameliorated either through medicine or by surgery.
 B. Sensorineural losses include hearing problems of a sensory or neural nature.
  1. Damage to hair cells or the eighth nerve results in sensorineural hearing loss.
  2. Common causes of sensorineural loss include: viral and bacterial infections, ototoxic drugs, excessive noise exposure, congenital anomalies, and head trauma.
  3. Since the physical appearance of the auditory canals is normal, losses of this type are frequently overlooked.
  4. Sensorineural hearing loss is almost always irreversible, and its only treatment is amplification and special education.

V. Assessment of Hearing Status
 A. History should include the following significant factors:
  1. Prenatal factors;
  2. Perinatal factors;
  3. Postnatal factors;

      4. Preschool history;

      5. Parental concern;

      6. Speech and language development.

    B. Physical examination should include evaluation of the ear canals and eardrums as well as a check for congenital anomalies of the ear, nose, and throat.

VI. Additional Assessment

    A. The suspect child under five years of age should be referred for evaluation.

    B. Audiometric screening is appropriate prior to referral for children five years of age and older.

VII. Referrals

    A. Criteria for referral include:

      1. Child has a history of any predisposing medical factors;

      2. Parents or physician are concerned about a hearing loss;

      3. Child has a speech or language delay;

      4. Child is otitis-prone.

    B. The child should be referred at the first suspicion of hearing impairment.

VIII. Summary

IMPORTANCE OF HEARING SCREENING

Hearing screening is an important part of a well-child checkup that is often overlooked. Since a hearing impairment affects the child's intellectual and social development, it is essential to determine whether or not a hearing impairment exists.

It is the purpose of this chapter to discuss the prevalence of hearing loss, the significance of the loss to the child, and the types of hearing losses and their respective prognoses.

PREVALENCE OF HEARING LOSS

Each year there are 3,000 to 4,000 profoundly deaf babies born in the United States. There are an additional 5,000 who have significant hearing impairments that require special education, perhaps accompanied by amplification, hearing aids, or special speech and hearing rehabilitation. And, no doubt, there are millions of other children with milder hearing losses whose problems are not noticed until they are identified by a school's screening program at grade one or perhaps not until grade five. As many as 15 percent of preschool children have mild to moderate hearing losses which are medically or surgically remediable if detected.

The prevalence of hearing loss increases in such special populations as Eskimos, Navajo Indians, and inner city children (among whom the prevalence may be as high as 20 percent). The prevalence is also higher among children with cleft palate, Down Syndrome, and craniofacial disorders.

SIGNIFICANCE OF HEARING LOSS TO THE CHILD

Undetected hearing problems can impair a child's intellectual development and create speech and language problems which can last a lifetime. The identification of hearing loss in children, to be sure, is not an easy task, and it typically requires an experienced audiologist to pinpoint the degree and severity of a hearing loss. In each case where misdiagnosis or mismanagement postpones the identification of a hearing loss, the irrecoverable loss in time adversely affects the child's intellectual and social growth.

Developmental delay and the communication habits of children are often associated with hearing loss, and the primary care physician should immediately consider the possibility of a hearing loss for any child exhibiting developmental delay. The physician should also bear in mind that the earlier the hearing loss is identified, the better the prognosis for the child.

Each year three to five percent of school-age children are identified as having mild to moderate hearing impairment. Often such a hearing impairment, even though it is considered mild, is sufficient to interfere with the child's scholastic growth.

CONDUCTIVE AND SENSORINEURAL HEARING LOSSES

There are two types of hearing losses: conductive and sensorineural.

Conductive hearing losses involve problems with the sound conduction mechanism or failure of the sound to reach the cochlea and organs of hearing; thus any sort of obstruction in the ear canal or the middle ear cavity that interferes with sound transmission is a conductive hearing loss. This type of hearing loss accounts for about 95 percent of hearing losses among infants and preschool-age children. The common causes of conductive hearing loss are foreign objects in the ear canal, debris in the external auditory canal, external otitis, any problems associated with tympanic membrane mobility (such as perforation or all the otitis media categories), and congenital anomalies (such as atresia of the external ear canal). Since a child who has conductive hearing loss has trouble receiving sound from the environment, it is likely that speech and language will not develop properly. It is also likely that the child will be developmentally delayed and will not progress at a normal rate. It is important to note that about 95 percent of all conductive-type hearing losses can be ameliorated either through medication or surgery.

The second major category of hearing loss, sensorineural hearing loss, includes sensory and neural problems. Damage to either the hair cells or the eighth nerve is considered to result in a sensorineural hearing loss. Common causes of sensorineural hearing loss include viral and bacterial infections, ototoxic drugs, excessive noise exposure, congenital anomalies, and head trauma. Since these conditions are also precursors of mental subnormality, the physician will find a higher prevalence of this type of loss among mentally retarded than among non-handicapped children of a similar age. Sensorineural hearing losses are commonly overlooked in children since the physical examination of these children appears absolutely normal. Their external auditory canals look normal; the tympanic membranes move normally to pneumatic otoscopy; and the physical otological examination will simply show nothing abnormal. It is especially important therefore, when examining a handicapped child or one who appears delayed, to investigate the possibility of sensorineural hearing loss.

With cochlea or eighth nerve damage, hearing losses cannot be treated medically or surgically. Since sensorineural hearing loss is nearly always irreversible, its only treatment is amplification and special education. So once again, the earlier this kind of hearing loss is identified, the sooner the task of rehabilitation (or habilitation in the case of small children who have never learned to speak or hear normally) can begin.

ASSESSMENT OF HEARING STATUS

Assessing the child's hearing status is an ongoing process since deafness or hearing loss can occur at any time in the child's life. There are various factors which have been associated with the onset of deafness that need to be addressed. These factors can be elicited through the history and/or through the mother's prenatal record and the child's birth record. These are listed in Table 6-1.

History-taking must include discussion with the parents, since one area of evaluation that cannot be overemphasized is that of parental concern. Is the parent concerned about the child's ability to hear? Some sample questions useful

TABLE 6-1   Hearing Checklist

Pregnancy History:
    Maternal illness, including
        Rubella_____
        Toxemia_____
        Diabetes_____
    Ototoxic drugs, including
        Streptomycin_____
        Neomycin_____
        Kanamycin_____
        Gentamicin_____
Birth History:
    Prematurity_____
    Hyperbilirubin_____
    Sepsis_____
Health History:
    Meningitis_____
    Sepsis_____
    Otitis media_____   Number of bouts*_____
Measles:
    Mumps_____
    Scarlet fever_____
    Whooping cough_____
Family History:
    Other relatives with significant
        hearing impairment from childhood_____
    Other relatives with congenital
        defect of ear, nose, throat_____
Medical Examination:
    Ear canals not clear_____
    Abnormal eardrum_____
    Congenital anomalies of
        Ear, nose, throat_____
        Mandible_____
        Head, face, neck_____

Conduct a *Hearing History,* using Table 6-2 to question the child's parents.

*Six or more confirmed bouts of otitis media are criteria for referral.

for children up to 12 months of age are included as Table 6-2. Questions for the older child usually are related to the child's speech and language development.

The speech and language development of the child is a good clue to the child's hearing function. A delay may signify a hearing loss. This, however, will be discussed in more depth in the chapter of this text entitled "Speech and Language Evaluation."

ADDITIONAL ASSESSMENT

As far as any additional assessment for hearing status, the following guidelines apply:

1. A child less than five years old should not be evaluated in the office. If a hearing problem is suspected, the child should be referred for an audiological examination.

2. For children five and six years of age, audiometric screening should be used prior to referral. (Screening with an audiometer and a tympanometer are described in Appendices A and B respectively.)

REFERRALS

There are four basic criteria to use when considering a referral for hearing loss in a child suspected of developmental delay. Refer the child if:

1. the history is positive of any of the predisposing medical factors (see Table 6-1);

TABLE 6-2 Hearing History*

4 Months

Hearing

1. Have you had any worry about your child's hearing?	YES	NO
2. When (s)he's sleeping in a quiet room does (s)he move and begin to wake up when there's a loud sound?	YES	NO
3. Does (s)he try to turn his or her head toward an interesting sound, or when his or her name is called?	YES	NO

6 Months

Hearing

1. Have you had any worry about your child's hearing?	YES	NO
2. When (s)he's sleeping in a quiet room, does (s)he move and begin to wake up when there's a loud sound?	YES	NO
3. Does (s)he turn his or her head toward an interesting sound or when his or her name is called?	YES	NO

8 Months

Hearing

1. Have you had any worry about your child's hearing?	YES	NO
2. When (s)he's sleeping in a quiet room, does (s)he move and begin to wake up when there's a loud sound?	YES	NO
3. Does (s)he turn his or her head directly toward an interesting sound or when his or her name is called?	YES	NO

10 Months

Hearing

1. Have you had any worry about your child's hearing?	YES	NO
2. When (s)he's sleeping in a quiet room, does (s)he move and begin to wake up when there's a loud sound?	YES	NO
3. Does (s)he turn his or her head directly toward an interesting sound or when his or her name is called?	YES	NO
4. Does (s)he enjoy ringing a bell or shaking a rattle?	YES	NO

11 Months

Hearing

1. Have you had any worry about your child's hearing?	YES	NO
2. When (s)he's sleeping in a quiet room, does (s)he move and begin to wake up when there's a loud sound?	YES	NO
3. Does (s)he turn his or her head directly toward an interesting sound or when his or her name is called?	YES	NO
4. Does (s)he try to imitate you when you make sounds?	YES	NO

12 Months

Hearing

1. Have you had any worry about your child's hearing?	YES	NO
2. When (s)he's sleeping in a quiet room, does (s)he move and begin to wake up when there's a loud sound?	YES	NO
3. Does (s)he turn his or her head directly toward an interesting sound or when his or her name is called?	YES	NO
4. Is (s)he beginning to repeat some of the sounds that you make?	YES	NO

*From Northern, J. L., and Downs, M. P. *Hearing in Children.* Baltimore: Williams and Wilkins, 1974.

2. the child is otitis-prone and has had six or more confirmed bouts of otitis media (Table 6-1);

3. the parents or physician are concerned that the child has a hearing problem (see Table 6-2);

4. the child has a speech and/or language delay (see the "Speech and Language Evaluation" chapter).

A child should be referred at the first suspicion of hearing impairment, whether that suspicion comes from the parent or whether it comes from the physician's contact with the child. Hearing loss is something which absolutely cannot wait for evaluation. It is something a child will not grow out of; when the physician first suspects a hearing problem, the child should be referred.

Referral should be to an audiologist or an otolaryngologist. If neither of these two individuals is available, the person responsible for testing hearing in the school system or the speech pathologist, who may be more knowledgeable than anyone else in the neighborhood about hearing impairment in children, should be considered.

Following appropriate referral, the physician should obtain information from the audiologist, otolaryngologist, or speech pathologist about the hearing status of that particular child. This report may come in the form of an audiogram, which is a graphic representation of hearing ability, but it more likely will be a letter describing the severity and degree (possibly even the etiology) of the hearing loss and the implications for the child's development.

SUMMARY

The habilitation or rehabilitation of any youngster who has a hearing impairment should be a combined effort of the primary care physician and the specialist who evaluates the hearing loss. Hearing loss is an insidious disease that is often very difficult to identify in children. Every primary care physician should be sensitive to this very important function in children who are suspected of having a developmental problem.

APPENDIX A

*Audiometric Screening**

The following is a step-by-step method for screening with an audiometer. Materials needed include an audiometer, a screening manual, a scoring form, and a quiet room.

SETTING UP THE AUDIOMETER

The audiometer must, of course, be plugged in and the power switch must be placed in the "on" position. The red and blue phone plugs must be properly connected to the red and blue audiometer outlets, and the tone switch must be turned to the "Off" or "Rev" position.

Next the operator should put the earphones on to see that the audiometer and both earphones are working for each frequency. The red phone is placed on the right ear. Then the following steps should be followed:

1. Frequency should be set at 1000 Hz, and the intensity dial should be set at 30 dB.
2. The output selector should be in the right (or red) position.
3. The interrupter switch should be pressed.
4. This procedure should be repeated for both 2000 and 4000 Hz frequencies.
5. Then the output selector should be moved to the left (or blue) position and the self-test should be repeated at 1000, 2000, and 4000 Hz frequencies.
6. Before beginning testing, the output selector should be returned to the right (or red) position.

INSTRUCTIONS TO THE CHILD

The child should be placed in a chair close to the audiometer, but in such a way that he or she cannot see either the face of the audiometer or the hands of the screener. The following are verbal instructions which the screener should give to the child:

Verbal Instructions	*Actions*
"We are going to play a listening game. In a few minutes, I'll let you wear the earphones like this."	The screener puts earphones on.
"You will hear some little sounds like a beep or a whistle in the earphones. You will hear something like this."	The screener gives example of audiometer tone by "beeping" or whistling for the child.
"Did you hear that? Everytime you hear the little whistle, you must put your hand up like this, and put it down quickly. When you hear the sound I make, put your hand up. Let's practice doing that."	THE SCREENER MUST SHOW HOW HE OR SHE WANTS THE HAND RAISED AND LOWERED; the screener whistles and demonstrates hand motion, then sees if child can respond alone 5 or 6 times as screener whistles or "beeps."
"Now listen to the whistle in the earphones. Put your hand up when you hear it, and then put your hand down quickly."	The screener holds the earphone 2 or 3 feet from the child. The intensity (loudness) dial is turned up to a high number

*Adapted from Frankenburg, W., Downs, M., and Kazuk, E., and Downs, M., Moor, P., and Frager, R. *The Denver Audiometric Screening Test,* University of Colorado Medical Center, 1973 and 1972.

"Listen carefully and put your hand up when you hear the little sound."

"Good for you!" (Each time child responds correctly, the screener nods and smiles.)

"No—listen carefully." (This response is if the child raises a hand when no sound is being presented.)

"Now it's your turn to wear the earphones and listen for the sounds."

and the interrupter switch is pressed so that the child can hear a tone.

The interrupter switch is pressed again (count one second—one-thousand-one) to see if child raises his or her hand. This process is repeated 5 or 6 times or until child understands completely what he or she is to do.

Following this verbal preparation, the earphones should be placed gently on the child so that the red earphone is on the right ear and the blue phone is on the left ear. The headband should be adjusted so that each earphone fits snugly against the ear; none of the child's hair should be between the ears and the earphones.

The screener should maintain a firm, positive attitude and show that the child's cooperation is expected.

SCREENING STEPS

The child's hearing should be tested (right ear first) at 1000, 2000, and 4000 Hz, all at 25 dB. Results should be recorded on the Audiometric Scoring Form.

AUDIOMETRIC SCORING FORM

DATE: TOTAL TEST RESULTS (Circle One): P   F   U

Frequency	Right Ear			Left Ear		
1000 Hz (25 dB)	P	F	U	P	F	U
2000 Hz (25 dB)	P	F	U	P	F	U
4000 Hz (25 dB)	P	F	U	P	F	U
COMMENTS:						

For screening at 1000 Hz, the following procedure should be used:

1. The first sound should be practiced (1000 Hz at 50 dB); then the output selector should be turned to the right ear.
2. The interrupter switch should be pressed for one second; the screener should use side vision to note the child's response, and should not look directly at the child.
3. Next, the intensity is changed to 35 dB and the interrupter switch is again pressed and response observed.
4. Then the intensity dial is set at 25 dB and the procedure is repeated.
5. The test is repeated at various time intervals until the child responds three times or fails to respond three times, whichever comes first.
6. The results are circled on the score sheet as "Pass," "Fail," or "Uncertain" for 1000 Hz, right ear.

Screening at 2000 and 4000 Hz are conducted and scored in the same manner as above, with the intensity dial set throughout at 25 dB.

Following this testing of the right ear, the output selector is moved to left (or blue) position and the test and scoring are then repeated.

HEARING SCREENING RESULTS

As puretones were presented to the child, the screener circled the appropriate ratings for both right and left ear and for 1000, 2000, and 4000 Hz (all at 25 dB). Next the screener records the overall test results on the top of the scoring form.

A "Pass" signifies that the child had three correct responses in both ears at all frequencies. A "Fail" signifies that the child had incorrect responses in one or more frequencies in either ear. And a score of "Uncertain" means either that the test was not completed, or that the screener was unsure of the child's responses.

If the screening test result was either a "Fail" or "Uncertain," the child should be rescreened within two weeks. If the child passes the second screening, he or she is considered to have adequate hearing.

TESTING THE YOUNG CHILD

The physician who wishes to test the hearing of young children should begin by becoming friendly with the parent and then talking to the child.

The physician should tell the child pleasantly but firmly what the child will do. It is unwise to ask the child if he or she is willing to cooperate, for the child may answer "no."

The young child may sit on the parent's lap, if that will increase his or her sense of security.

The screener should be prepared to move to another method if the child becomes restless. If the child objects to the earphone placed over the head, the parent can hold the earphone to the child's ear. In such a case, careful instruction needs to be given to the parent to assure the correct placement of the earphone and to assure that the ear canal is not occluded by too much pressure.

When testing a child under five years of age, it is necessary to maintain interest with something that is fun for the child; even older children may not be interested in simply raising a hand when the tone is heard. A child whose mental age seems lower than five years should be treated as if he or she were younger, regardless of actual age.

Simple toys may help maintain a child's interest and cooperation in the screening test. Instead of being asked to raise one hand, the child may be taught to respond to tones by building a tower of blocks, adding one block for each tone heard, or by placing: a marble or pellet in a box or bottle; colored rings on a peg; a small wooden peg in a pegboard; small cars, trucks, etc., in a garage; or animals in a barnyard at each tone.

All that is necessary is that the child understand what is wanted and responds consistently so the screener knows the test tones have been heard. The screener can switch from one kind of play to another, if that is necessary to maintain the child's attention, but with each change in play the child should be reminded to respond only when he or she hears the tone.

If the child refuses to cooperate with the screener, the parent can be asked to practice at home with the child so he or she will know what to do during the next screening test. The parents can blow a whistle or horn or make some other noise and get the child to respond appropriately. After a week or so of practice, the screening should be repeated.

APPENDIX B

*Tympanometry Screening**

IMPORTANCE OF TYMPANOMETRY

Tympanometry is becoming a widely-used method of evaluating the physiological functions of the middle ear; its sensitivity in detecting even very mild pathologic conditions of the middle ear makes it especially valuable for use with children.

Otologists stress that pneumatic otoscopy is absolutely necessary to identify the presence of middle ear disease, yet only one-fourth of all physicians use the pneumatic otoscope. Most physicians who do use otoscopy to visually examine the tympanic membrane do so with varying degrees of success. A recent study of the accuracy of otoscopic diagnoses found that because accurate otoscopy requires skill and experience, 15 to 20 percent of middle ear effusions in children under three years of age were missed clinically.

Problems encountered in otoscopy include difficulty in visualizing the tympanic membrane, the necessity for removal of cerumen prior to examination, and the unwillingness of some children to cooperate with the otoscopic examination.

Tympanometry is best defined as electronic pneumatic otoscopy. It resolves many of the disadvantages of conventional audiology and otologic assessment, since it requires only passive cooperation from children and does not depend on overt responses. In addition, it does not require the removal of the cerumen from the ear, since total visualization of the tympanic membrane is not necessary.

Many pediatricians are beginning to realize that tympanometry, in combination with audiometry, medical history and physical examination, constitutes the best approach to detecting middle ear disease and hearing impairment in children.

HOW TYMPANOMETRY WORKS

Tympanometry determines the compliance (or mobility) of the tympanic membrane and middle ear system by measuring reflected sound energy. This compliance measurement is obtained at specific air pressures created in a hermetically sealed external ear canal.

The probe tip, which is sealed in the external ear canal, has three small holes: the first emits a 220 Hz probe tone; the second permits the manipulation of air pressure by an external pump; and the third utilizes a microphone which measures the intensity of the probe tone as it is reflected by the patient's tympanic membrane.

Compliance of the tympanic membrane is of particular clinical significance, since most pathological conditions involving the membrane or middle ear cavity influence the mobility of the tympanic membrane. Tympanometry precisely measures compliance within a range of from +200 to −400 mm H_2O, relative to atmospheric air pressure.

Maximum compliance of the membrane occurs when the air pressure in the external ear canal equals the pressure in the middle ear. Patients who have intact tympanic membranes, normal middle ear function, and adequate Eustachian tube function show maximum compliance of the tympanic membrane at atmospheric air pressure.

OTITIS MEDIA

Accurate measurement of middle ear pressure may provide significant clinical information relative to otitis media. When the process of aeration in the middle ear is halted during obstruction of the Eustachian tube, the now-static air in the middle ear space is absorbed, and negative air pressure is produced in the middle ear space, ultimately causing the transudation of fluid and retraction of the tympanic membrane. Early identification of negative middle ear pressure may permit the physician to practice preventive medicine by avoiding middle ear effusion and concomitant hearing loss.

HEARING TESTS

Screening for hearing loss and the identification of ear disease are two separate objectives. Tympanometry is quite sensitive in the accurate identification of middle ear problems, but a threshold hearing test is absolutely necessary to identify possible hearing loss. Therefore, the use of tympanometry does not preclude the necessity of a hearing test.

Numerous studies have been performed

---

*Adapted in part from Northern J., and Downs, M. *Hearing in Children*. Baltimore: Williams and Wilkins Co., 1974.

which indicate that audiometric hearing levels do not necessarily identify middle ear pathology. For example, Cohen and Sade studied 408 ears with serous otitis media in 1972. They found that 50 percent of those ears would have been passed as "normal" on school hearing tests conducted at the accepted screening hearing level of 25 dB HTL. Clearly, puretone audiometric screening is insufficient and is not the technique of choice for the identification of ear disease. However, the majority of school systems in this country continue to use audiometric screening under the misguided assumption that children will be appropriately referred for medical evaluation and treatment.

TYMPANOMETRY AND HANDICAPPED CHILDREN

Tympanometry has proven valuable in the auditory evaluation of special-population children who are at high risk of developing chronic middle ear disease. These include: children of particular ethnic groups such as American Indians and American Eskimos; children who are difficult to test, such as the retarded, developmentally delayed, deaf, deaf-blind, and multiply handicapped; and groups in which a high incidence of middle ear disease may be expected, such as patients with cleft lip and palate, Down Syndrome, allergies, or cranial-facial or skeletal disorders.

IMPEDANCE AUDIOMETRY

The test battery for impedance audiometry includes not only tympanometry, but also static compliance and acoustic reflex threshold measurement. Each of these procedures can provide significant information; however, their diagnostic capabilities are strengthened when results from the three procedures are considered together.

The following summarizes the applications of impedance audiometry in children. Tympanometry provides:

1. an objective measurement of tympanic membrane mobility;
2. a measurement of middle ear pressure;
3. identification of tympanic membrane perforations;

4. confirmation of ventilation tubes potency in the tympanic membrane; and
5. an estimate of static compliance.

Static compliance provides a differentiation of middle ear fixation from disarticulation. Acoustic reflex threshold provides:

1. an objective measurement of loudness requirement;
2. validation of nonorganic and conductive hearing loss;
3. a differential diagnosis of conductive hearing loss; and
4. an objective inference of hearing sensitivy.

SUMMARY

There is little question that under proper circumstances and when time permits, the most thorough evaluation of auditory problems is accomplished through the use of otoscopic examination, auditory threshold testing, and impedance audiometry. However, when less-than-optimal conditions exist, or when a well-qualified otoscopic examiner is unavailable, tympanometry is undoubtedly the most sensitive indicator of middle ear disease. It has also proven a useful supplement to traditional diagnostic techniques.

BIBLIOGRAPHY

Downs, M. P. Hearing loss: Definition, epidemiology, and prevention. *Public Health Reviews,* 1973, *4* (3), 255–277.

Downs, M. P. Auditory screening. *Otolaryngology Clinics of North America,* 1978, *11,* 611–629.

Harfard, E. R., Bess, F. H., Bluestone, C. D., and Klein, J. O. (Eds.). *Impedance screening for middle ear disease in children.* New York: Grune and Stratton, 1977.

Northern, J. L. Advanced techniques for measuring middle ear function. *Pediatrics,* 1978, *61,* 761–767.

Northern, J. L. (Ed.). *Hearing disorders.* Boston: Little, Brown and Co., 1976.

Northern, J. L., and Downs, M. P. *Hearing in children.* Baltimore: Williams and Wilkins, second edition, 1978.

Steward, J. M., Peterson, R. A., Abroms, I. F., Holmes, L. B., and Boyle, P. Medical and psychological evaluation. In B. Jaffe (Ed.), *Hearing loss in children.* Baltimore: University Park Press, 1977.

Chapter 7

Goal
To develop skills in the assessment of speech and language development, in the treatment of mild language problems, and in making appropriate referrals to a speech pathologist.

Objectives
At the end of this chapter, the physician should be able to:

- describe the communication process model and how it relates to language development in children;
- identify six causes of language delay;
- assess a child for language development with an age-appropriate test;
- identify children who need a home stimulation program or referral to a speech pathologist;
- refer children appropriately to a speech pathologist.

SPEECH AND LANGUAGE EVALUATION

By
FLORENCE BERMAN BLAGER, Ph.D.

I. Importance of Speech and Language Development
Speech and language development are indicators of a child's over-all development, since they involve the cognitive, sensorimotor, psychological, emotional, and environmental systems.

II. Conceptual Language Development Model
   A. Speech and language skills should occur in developmental sequences.
   B. Any delay should be looked upon as a symptom for which there may be an underlying cause or causes.
   C. Early intervention will generally yield the best results.
   D. Effective communication requires reception of sound, association of meanings, and expression of thought; language should be thought of as encompassing these three processes.

III. Age of Language Development
   A. By the age of one year, normal children have obtained at least one first spoken word.
   B. Development of word sequences equivalent to chronological age is a minimal expectation of a young child's expressive language.

IV. Causes of Delay
   A. Environmental causes of language delay can include economic deprivation, family pressure, or bilingualism.
   B. Emotional problems, either the child's or a parent's, can interfere with normal language development.
   C. Even minor hearing losses can slow language acquisition.
   D. Mental retardation delays the acquisition of language skills.
   E. Birth defects may result in ongoing speech and language problems.
   F. Brain damage, from either trauma or disease, can interfere with appropriate development of speech.
   G. Difficulties with processing language also slow language acquisition.

V. Diagnostic Evaluation
   A. The first step in diagnostic evaluation is review of the medical history.
   B. The second is the physician's review of the speech and language portion of the medical examination.
   C. Questions which the physician should answer are as follows:
      1. Does the child listen? (Reception)
      2. Does the child understand what is said? (Comprehension)
      3. Does the child talk? (Expression)
      4. If the child does not talk, does he or she pantomime, show frustration at being asked to repeat, etc.?
      5. Does the child communicate differently with family members than with the physician?
   D. Because a child is intact in one language process does not mean that the other processes are intact.

VI. Administration of Language Tests
    A. Speech and language tests are usually standardized to separate the infant and toddler (up to three years) from the preschool-age child (three to six years).
    B. The Bzoch-League Receptive-Expressive Emergent Language Scale (REEL) is used for children up to three years of age and delineates speech and language acquisition in small age increments by questioning a parent.
    C. The REEL also helps evaluate how a child attends to and understands speech and language, apart from how the child produces speech and language.

VII. Administration of the REEL
    A. Questions should be asked of a parent in a broad manner; if the response does not answer specific questions, questions can be asked more directly.
    B. Receptive language questions are presented first, beginning at the child's chronological age level.
    C. The ceiling is the highest age category in which at least two pluses are recorded; a plus/minus counts as a plus only when there are two other pluses in the age category, or when the next higher age category is passed.
    D. Expressive questioning begins at the receptive language ceiling.
    E. Receptive and Expressive Languages Ages are recorded on the front of the test form; a Combined Language Age should not be computed.

VIII. Administration of the Peabody
    A. The Peabody is designed for children between three and six years of age; it tests single word receptive vocabulary.
    B. Seven rules for administering the Peabody are as follows:
        1. The test should be given in a quiet room;
        2. The child's choice, whether right or wrong, should be praised;
        3. Test words can be repeated, but not used in sentences; articles should not be used before nouns;
        4. The child should be encouraged to make a response;
        5. The child should be encouraged to look at all of the pictures;
        6. The child's final response should be recorded;
        7. Additional techniques (suggested in the Peabody manual) can be used with handicapped children.
    C. Testing begins at the child's chronological age on test Form A; the number of the picture which the child selected is recorded, and a slash is made through the accompanying symbol if the choice was wrong.
    D. The basal is the lowest of eight correct responses in a row; if the child makes an error before eight correct responses have been recorded, testing must continue backward from the starting point.
    E. The ceiling is the highest item when there have been six errors out of eight consecutive responses; this is found by beginning at the child's first error.
    F. The ceiling is recorded on the front of the score sheet; then the number of errors made is subtracted to obtain a raw score; and a mental age is extrapolated from the Peabody manual.
    G. Since the Peabody is not a valid I.Q. test, the child's I.Q. should not be computed.
    H. The administrator records first the ceiling, then the total number of errors; when the errors are subtracted from the ceiling, the raw score is recorded on the test form.
    I. Page 12 of the Peabody manual contains a table that provides the mental age equivalents of raw scores; this mental age is also written on the text form.

IX. Interpreting Language Test Results
 A. The Receptive and Expressive Language Ages on the REEL and the Mental Age on the Peabody are compared to the child's chronological age on Table 7–6.
 B. Table 7–6 indicates whether the amount of delay is a matter for concern or an indication for referral.
XI. Intervention and Referral
 A. Each child with a language delay should have a hearing test by an audiologist or trained speech pathologist.
 B. If the delay seems to stem from lack of adequate home stimulation, the physician can undertake one stimulation goal per visit with the parent.
 C. If the delay continues or worsens despite stimulation efforts, the child should be referred to a speech pathologist.
 D. When a delay is due to minimal parental depression, the physician can attempt counseling; if the depression is more serious, the parent should be referred for treatment.
 E. The child with a language delay due to a birth defect should be referred to a special clinic as early as possible.
 F. When language delays result from brain damage, referral procedures vary, depending upon the child's problems.
XII. Referral Procedures
 A. The physician should provide information at the time of referral, including test results, observations, and suspicions.
 B. The physician should request a report covering the significance and causes of a delay as well as recommendations for intervention.
 C. When concerned, the physician should always refer.
 D. The physician should establish a community resource list to speed referrals when they become necessary.
XIII. Articulation
 A. Evaluation of articulation requires special training and practice.
 B. Each physician's office should have trained personnel available to conduct articulation evaluations.
XIV. Summary

IMPORTANCE OF SPEECH AND LANGUAGE DEVELOPMENT

Speech and language are important indicators of a child's overall development. They are sensitive to delay or damage in other systems precisely because they involve other systems—the cognitive, sensorimotor, psychological, emotional, and environmental systems.

The purpose of this chapter is to provide an approach to help the physician detect speech and language delays. The information will include: a conceptual model of the speech and language process; milestones of emerging language; an observational guide for use during examination of the child; significant points to be established in the medical history; the use of specific tests; and finally, guidelines as to when the physician should refer the child, or when the physician should attempt direct intervention.

CONCEPTUAL LANGUAGE DEVELOPMENT MODEL

Talking is normal, and not talking is not. While this may seem obvious, too often a child with delayed speech is treated as if speech will begin when the child is ready. Few physicians, confronted by a boy who is old enough to walk but who isn't, would comfort the mother by saying, "Well, he'll walk when he's

TABLE 7-1   Clinical Model of Human Communication*

	Reception	*Comprehension*	*Expression*
Level III	Comprehension ———————→	Conceptual ———————→	Intentional
Level II	Perception ———————————→	Automatic ————————→	Spontaneous
Level I	Sensation ————————————→	Reflexive ————————→	Expletive

*Derived from Wepman, Osgood, Carrow, and Blager

ready." It is easy to think of walking as a normal developmental action; if it does not occur by a more or less expected time, it serves as an indicator that something might be wrong.

Speech and language are similar skills, with normal developmental sequences. They should occur within a certain range of time, and should not be dismissed as if the child will simply begin talking when ready. The speech or language delay should be looked upon as a symptom for which there may well be some underlying cause or a combination of causes. Most of these causes will respond appreciably to intervention, and as in most problems, the earlier the needed intervention is started, the more swiftly progress will occur.

In evaluating language, it is helpful to think of all the processes involved. This is particularly true of children with unintelligible speech who seem to understand what is said to them, or of children who speak clearly and yet need a great deal of explaining before they understand a task.

Table 7-1 contains three columns. One column is labeled reception, one, comprehension, and the third, expression. Reception refers to receiving sound through the ears (how it is heard and perceived). Comprehension refers to applying meaning to the sound heard, and using that meaning in thinking. Expression refers to using that sound or word in spoken, written, or other forms of language.

The model also divides language into three levels. Level I is the reflexive level. A child who accidentally bumps into a stove and says "Uh-Oh!" will quickly hear that sound used by the mother as a warning. Soon "Uh-Oh!" will come to mean that there is danger imminent and that the child should be careful.

Level II, the next level higher, is automatic language. This is language that eventually becomes what the name describes—it is used without much conscious thought. Exchanges such as, "How are you?" and, "Fine, thank you," like the days of the week or the months of the year, are all examples of automatic language.

Level III, the highest level, is the level of comprehension and conceptualization. It is language used in understanding and communicating.

AGE OF LANGUAGE DEVELOPMENT

The sequence of language development is usually from sounds to babbling to jargon. First the child begins to make individual sounds, then to connect strings of sounds together with an intonation pattern that has the sound of language, but is conducted without real words. All this takes place before one year of age.

As shown in Table 7-2, the majority of children speak their first word by 12 months of age. Only two percent are over 24 months of age when their first word is spoken. Word sequences start at two years of age for 89 percent of all children.

A good rule of thumb is that until four or five years of age, a child should be

TABLE 7-2   Development of Speech*

	Age	%
Single Words	9–12 Months	66%
	12 Months	73%
	Before 8 Months	7%
	Over 24 Months	2%
Word Sequences	18 Months	40%
	17–24 Months	67%
	24 Months	89%
	Before 12 Months	9%

*From M. E. Morley

using word sequences at least equivalent to age. That is, at one year the child should be using one-word sequences (ball, doggie, mama). At two years, the child should speak in two-word sequences (go now, more cookie). At three years, the listener should hear three-word sequences; and so forth, up to four or five years of age. A word-per-year is a good minimal expectation of a child's expressive language in these early years.

This is the way that language develops in most children. What are the factors that can cause delays in this expected sequence?

CAUSES OF DELAY

The cause of language delay are explored in Table 7–3 from the more extrinsic to the more intrinsic. The causes include: environmental factors; emotional problems; hearing losses; mental retardation; birth defects; brain damage; and language-processing difficulties.

The first cause of language delay is environmental. Children who talk early and well usually grow up in families that talk well. Children from families that do not speak well usually develop speech and language at a slower rate. Specific environmental problems can include: deprivation, family pressure, or bilingualism. Deprivation among children from low socioeconomic levels can result in delayed acquisition of speech and language. Family pressure, another environmental factor, can result in stuttering. The high-achieving family may impose too much pressure on a speech system in these early

TABLE 7-3   Causes of Speech and Language Problems

Cause	*Effect on Speech and Language Development*
1. Environmental	
a. Low socioeconomic level	a. Delayed
b. Family pressure	b. Stuttering
c. Nonverbal family	c. Delayed acquisition of language
d. Bilingual home	d. Delayed acquisition of language structure
2. Emotional	
a. Depressed mother	a. Delayed acquisition
b. Seriously disturbed parent	b. Delayed or distorted development
c. Seriously disturbed child	c. Delayed or distorted development
3. Hearing Problems	
a. Congenital	a. Delayed or permanently impaired
b. Acquired	b. Delayed or permanently impaired
4. Developmental Delay	
a. Slow development	a. Delayed development
b. Low, but within average development	b. Delayed development
c. Mental retardation	c. Significantly delayed development
5. Birth Defects	
a. Cleft palate	a. Delayed and impaired development
b. Down Syndrome	b. Lower than other developmental areas
6. Brain Damage	
a. Neuromuscular damage	a. Interference with sucking, swallowing, chewing; later, speech and articulation problems such as dysarthria
b. Sensorimotor problems	b. Interference with sucking, swallowing; later, articulation problems such as dyspraxia
c. Cerebral palsy	c. Significant interference with respiration, feeding; articulation problems may have components of dysarthria and dyspraxia
d. Perceptual problems	d. Difficulty with sound discrimination, understanding spoken language, symbolization, generating verbal concepts; later, in school, learning disabilities

years, and the result can be dysfluency. Bilingualism during the years a child is first learning to talk can delay acquisition of language. If the child is bright, he or she will come through this period of early confusion and develop two intact language systems. Sometimes it is not bilingualism alone that is the impeding factor. It is often compounded by environmental deprivation from low socioeconomic levels.

The next cause of language delay is an emotional problem—of either the parent or the child. A mother who is depressed may be able to bathe or feed the child, but may not be able to talk very much to that child. The mother who is seriously emotionally disturbed can cause even more damage to the developing speech and language of the child. The child who is withdrawn and shows little response to nurturing may be a child with severe emotional problems; these problems will interfere with normal speech and language development.

Hearing problems, which may be either congenital or acquired, can lead to language delay. Even mild losses from chronic otitis media, particularly when the losses occur before two years of age, can interfere with speech and language development. Such losses can also result in delays in learning at school.

Developmental delays are another cause of slow language development. The child who is slow in developing will have delayed speech and language skills as well. If the delay is more severe and the child is retarded, speech and language skills will certainly be retarded. Sometimes, speech itself may be rather fluent, but the limited conceptual level of the language will reflect mental retardation.

Language delays can also result from birth defects. Cleft palate and Down Syndrome are not merely factors that can cause speech and language delays. These are examples of congenital problems that result in ongoing speech and language problems.

Brain damage may also affect the acquisition of speech and language skills. Brain damage may occur prenatally, postnatally, or perinatally, or it may occur from trauma or disease. The result can be sensorimotor or neuromotor damage that interferes with the development of early sucking, swallowing, or chewing responses. This can lead to articulation problems such as inconsistent patterning of sounds (apraxia), or more serious consistent articulation problems (dysarthria). More severe brain damage can result in cerebral palsy, with accompanying speech and language problems.

There may also be problems in language processing. As presented in the conceptual model of language, although hearing is intact a child may have difficulty understanding what is said, and/or there may be difficulty in finding the words with which to respond. These language processing problems may be severe enough to result in childhood aphasia, or may be subtle enough to result in school learning problems.

DIAGNOSTIC EVALUATION

This chapter thus far has examined: a conceptual model of language that is a framework in understanding speech and language problems; the ages when emerging language should occur; and causative factors that interfere with normal speech and language development.

The following discussion will focus on the effect of problem areas on speech and language development, and how the physician can diagnose and treat the speech and language problems that may be present.

In diagnosing speech and language problems, the physician should:

1. review the medical history, particularly the speech and language portions;
2. review the speech and language portion of the medical examination;
3. administer language tests;
4. evaluate significant delays;
5. intervene when that is necessary;
6. refer the child to specialists when appropriate.

The first step is for the physician to review the medical history. If any of the causative factors have appeared, if any delays have been found through the use of screening tests, or if the examiner's observations have indicated that communication is difficult for the child, the physician should explore more thoroughly the speech and language portion of the medical history shown in Table 7-4. This includes both the developmental milestones and the systems review.

The next step is for the physician to review the speech and language portion of the medical examination more thoroughly. This section is shown in Table 7-5. It contains a series of questions for the physician to answer while examining the child, and is one of the most important components of the evaluation.

The questions to be answered by the physician on Table 7-5 are based on the same three components of reception (listening), comprehension (understanding), and expression (talking) presented in Table 7-1.

During the examination of a child, the physician should ask him- or herself the following questions.

First, does the child listen? The physician should note whether or not the child looks at the person who is speaking, and whether the child responds to his or her own name.

Second, does the child understand what is said? The physician can answer this question by observing whether the child follows directions. For example, when addressed, the child may look puzzled unless the words are accompanied by gestures which make the meaning clear, unless the language is simplified, or unless the speaker either speaks more loudly or more slowly than normal.

Third, does the child talk? Do the sounds or words the child uses resemble real words? For example, it is very good when a child who is beginning to talk says "buh" for ball or baby or bottle. It is less good if the child says "guh" for the same words. It is good for the child to say "kaka" for cookie or cracker; it is very bad for the child to say "glee" for those words. This is because "buh" uses a sound of the intended word, and can evolve into the whole word when the child's articulatory control matures. "Glee" does not use any of the sounds of cookie or cracker, and indicates that speech may not mature into the intended word. The physician should note whether the child's speech is understandable, if talking is related to the situation, and whether the child shows any unnecessary mouth movements or drooling.

TABLE 7-4 Medical History

Developmental Milestones–Speech and Language

Language:	Age Expected:
Babbles to self	2 months
Repeats sounds others make	9 months
Says mama or dada appropriately	10 to 12 months
Uses first words with meaning	12 months
Says three single words	12 months
Repeats words others say	18 months
Uses sentences	24 months
Combines different words in phrases	36 months

Systems Review–Speech and Language

1. Has your child ever had any problems swallowing, chewing, or drooling?
2. Has your child ever been evaluated or received therapy for speech, language, perceptual, or psychological problems?
3. Do you have any concerns about your child's speech and language? If so, what are they?
4. If so, when did you first become concerned about the speech and language development?
5. Do any other members of your family have problems in this area (delayed speech, reading problems, learning problems, stuttering, etc.)?
6. Do you speak more than one language in your home?
7. Has your child's hearing ever been questioned or tested?

TABLE 7-5　Speech and Language Examination

---

1. Reception—*Does the child listen?*
   Attentive to speech_____; Looks at person speaking_____;
   Responds to name_____.
2. Comprehension—*Does the child understand what is said?*
   Follows directions_____; Looks puzzled unless examiner: uses gestures_____; simplifies what is said_____; speaks slowly_____; speaks loudly_____.
3. Expression—*Does the child talk?*
   Sounds resemble words_____; Speech is understandable_____;
   Talking is related to the situation_____; Imitates sounds, but can't produce them spontaneously _____.
4. Expression—*What if the child doesn't talk?*
   Pantomimes_____; Shows frustration if asked to repeat_____;
   Makes sounds spontaneously, but can't imitate_____; Imitates sounds, but can't produce them spontaneously_____.
5. *Does the child communicate differently with family members than with the physician?*
   More or less infantile_____; More or less clear_____; More or less talkative_____; No observable differences_____.

Fourth, what if the child doesn't talk? Perhaps a child pantomimes instead of attempting speech. Perhaps the child shows frustration if asked to repeat a phrase. Or perhaps the child may be able to imitate the speaker, but may seem unable to produce sounds spontaneously.

And fifth, does the child communicate differently with family members than with the examiner? The physician may note that a child sounds more infantile when talking to the mother in the waiting room than to the physician during the examination. Perhaps the child talks freely with the mother but totally "clams up" during an examination. Note whether the child's speech sounds more clear, less clear, or the same when the child talks with the parent as contrasted with when the child talks with the physician.

The child should be observed with these points in mind. During the examination or testing of the child, the physician should remember the basic questions of how well the child listens, understands, and talks. The physician should be aware of anything special done with the child to improve communication. Because a child is intact in one language process does not mean that the other processes are intact. If any aspect of communication is arduous for the child, the evaluator, or the parent, then the physician should be suspicious of possible language problems.

ADMINISTRATION OF LANGUAGE TESTS

The next step is for the physician to administer language tests. Speech and language tests are usually standardized to separate the infant and toddler (up to three years) from the preschool child (from three to six years). The two tests presented here reflect this age division.

The first, the Bzoch-League Receptive-Expressive Emergent Language Scale (known as the REEL), is used for children up to three years of age. The second, the Peabody Picture Vocabulary Test, can be used for children between three and six years of age.

The REEL is a questionnaire which is not difficult to administer. Since young children will not always perform upon demand, the REEL questionnaire helps supplement observations of speech and language skills by having someone who knows the child well report speech and language development. It delineates speech and language acquisition by small age increments. This is very important, particularly in the early years, for a two-month delay of language in the life of a 12-month-old is much more significant than a two-month delay in the life of a six-year-old. Another strength of the REEL is that it separates receptive from expressive language. It helps evaluate how the child *attends to* and understands speech and language, apart from how the child *produces* speech and language. If the child has no problems, it can be administered in about three minutes. If the child does have delays, it will take about 10 minutes to explore the examples requested from the parents.

ADMINISTRATION OF THE REEL*

The REEL consists of a manual and a scoring form. It is administered by interviewing the parent or someone who knows the child well enough to answer the questions. These questions, which are divided into age categories, should initially be asked in a broad manner. For example, for a child two-and-one-half months of age, receptive questions R7 to R9 would be asked; the administrator might first ask, "How does Jamie respond when you talk to him?" Then, if the parent's response did not answer each specific item in the age category, the test administrator could ask the questions more directly. For question R7, for example, a more direct question would be, "Does he turn his head toward your face when you talk to him?"

Questions should not be posed in such a way that the parent believes the answer should be "yes." Instead, the administrator should give the impression that it does not really matter whether a "yes" or a "no" answer is given. Sometimes the word "yet" can be added at the end of a question, implying that both the administrator and the parent know the behavior is coming, but that it will take a little longer. If the administrator is unsure of the parent's answer, two examples of the behavior can be requested. The important point to remember is that broad questions should be asked first, so that a general impression of the child's language performance can be formed before specific details are suggested to the parent.

When the parent indicates that the child can perform an item, a plus (+) is

recorded. When the parent says that the child cannot perform an item, a minus (−) is recorded. If the parent says the child only sometimes performs an item, a plus/minus (±) is recorded.

The receptive language questions, on the left side of the scoring form, should be presented first. Normally, the test administrator should begin asking questions at the age level that corresponds to the child's chronological age. This age is computed on the front of the scoring form in the same manner as demonstrated earlier for computing ages for developmental screening tests. This is done by subtracting the child's birthdate from the date of administration of the test. Beginning questioning at the level of the child's chronological age will pose no problems when dealing with a child whose speech and language development are relatively normal. However, for a delayed child, the chronological age level may be too high. For this reason, some experienced test administrators, having seen a child before the test and believing that there is a speech and language delay, may begin their questioning at an age level lower than chronological age. In other words, they may begin at the age level where the child appears to be functioning. However, persons who have not had much experience in administering the REEL will find it best to begin at the recommended age level.

The next step is to find the child's ceiling, which is the highest age category in which the child receives at least two pluses. For example, during receptive questioning, if a child receives two pluses in the 22- to 24-month age category, and then receives two minuses in the 24- to 27-month age category, the receptive ceiling is 24 months. The child is given credit for the top of the highest age category obtained. In other words, the child whose ceiling is in the 22- to 24-month receptive age category receives a 24-month score for receptive language. To reiterate, each child is given credit for an entire age-range grouping when any two of the three items in that grouping have been scored as a plus.

The only exception to the require-

---

*Adapted from Bzoch, Kenneth, R., and League, Richard, *Assessing Language Skills in Infancy.* University Park Press: Baltimore, 1971.

ment that a minimum of two pluses be present in an age category to establish a ceiling involves the plus/minus. A plus/minus counts as a plus when the child receives two additional pluses in that age category; then he or she is considered to have passed to the next age level. However, if a child receives a plus, a minus, and a plus/minus, he or she is considered to have passed the age category only if the next higher age interval is passed. If the two needed pluses in the next age category are not obtained, the previous plus, minus, and plus/minus must be scored as a fail.

Once the child's receptive ceiling has been determined, it is recorded as the Receptive Language Age on the front of the scoring form. Then, the Expressive Language questions on the right-hand side of the scoring form should be asked. Expressive questioning begins not at the child's chronological age, but at the child's Receptive Language Age. With expressive, as receptive questioning, the test administrator scores either upward or downward through the age levels until the child's ceiling—two pluses in an age category before two minuses in the next highest age category—is found. When this has been obtained, the top age the child received expressively should be written onto the front of the scoring form in the blank marked Expressive Language Age.

These should not be combined into the Combined Language Age, as the REEL manual indicates. Instead, it is vital to look at receptive and expressive language ages separately in comparison with the child's chronological age.

ADMINISTRATION OF THE PEABODY*

The Peabody Picture Vocabulary Test is designed for children whose functional language development is between three and six years of age. It tests a child's strength in language by testing single word receptive vocabulary. It pro-

vides pictures to test if the child comprehends a word's meaning, gives the child a limited number of possibilities from which to select, and does not require that the child verbalize an answer—which may be difficult for children with some kinds of handicaps. The Peabody consists of a manual, two scoring forms, and a book of picture plates containing four pictures to the page.

Three trial plates—Examples A, B, and C—have been included for use prior to administration of the Peabody to ensure that the child being tested understands what he or she is supposed to do. The test is introduced by showing Example A and saying to the child, "I want to play a picture game with you. See all the pictures on this page. I'll say a word, and then I want you to put your finger on the picture of the word I've said. Let's try one. Put your finger on 'Bed.'" When the child responds correctly, the administrator says, "Good! Now try another one." This procedure is repeated with each example until the test administrator is sure the child understands what is required.

There are seven important rules for administering the Peabody. They are as follows:

1. The test should be given in a quiet room that is free from distractions.
2. The child should be encouraged by praise for each choice—whether the choice was right or wrong. The administrator can say, "Good," or "You're doing fine," or "Good job;" however, some children will know when praise is unearned. If a child asks, "Did I get that one right?" the administrator can respond, "That was a good answer."
3. The test words can be repeated more than once, if necessary, but they cannot be used in a sentence for the child. Most of the test words are in the singular; they must not be converted to the plural, for this may give the child a clue. In addition, the administrator must not say "the," "a," or "an" before a word, since use of an article before the test word can provide a clue to the child that the word is a noun.
4. If a child is slow in making a choice, he or she can be encouraged to make a

---

*Adapted from Dunn, Loyd M., *Peabody Picture Vocabulary Test Manual*. American Guidance Service, Inc.: Circle Pines, Minnesota, 1965.

choice. There is no provision for recording "no response" or "don't know" on the test; neither is there any penalty for guessing.

5. Some children, especially those who are very young, may point repeatedly to one corner on plate after plate. With such children, the administrator must frequently say, "Be sure to look carefully at all four of the pictures." If the child persists in pointing in a pattern, the test word can be given while the administrator points and says, "Look at this one, and this one, and this one, and this one."

6. When the child spontaneously changes his or her choice, the final response should be recorded. If the child points to two pictures at once, he or she can be asked to point again.

7. For young or handicapped children, some additional techniques can be used. For example, a young child may respond best by being asked to "put a block on the right picture." The Peabody manual contains additional suggestions for working with children who have severe cerebral palsy, and so on.

Testing is begun with Form A. (Two forms are provided; Form B is for use only when a child is being re-tested at a later time.) The child's age is calculated on the front of Form A. This procedure is described on page 9 of the Peabody manual, and consists of subtracting the child's birthdate from the date of testing. When the child's age has been computed, the administrator turns to page 2 inside the test form to see suggested starting points based on the age of the child. If a child is suspected of delayed development, the test administrator can drop back to what is believed to be the functional age. However, it is probably best for persons unfamiliar with the Peabody to begin at the plate recommended on the test form.

When scoring, the number of the picture which the child selected is recorded in the appropriate blank. If the child made an incorrect response, the administrator also makes a slash through the symbol—the star, circle, square, cross, triangle, and so forth—next to the blank

for that plate. Using the number of the picture the child selected will help the administrator re-check scoring at the end, and shows if the child is picking pictures in a random pattern. The slash through the symbols to the right aids in counting the number of errors the child has made. The symbols—the stars, circles, triangles, and so forth—are repeated every eight plates, and were designed to speed counting to find the basal and the ceiling.

The basal is the lowest of eight correct responses in a row. To establish the basal, the administrator starts at the plate indicated for the child's age and works upward until the child makes an error. If there have been eight consecutive correct responses in a row before that first error, the starting point is the basal. More frequently (especially with delayed children), a child will begin to work forward correctly, but will miss one item before eight correct responses in a row have been recorded. For example, if the child has four correct responses, but the fifth response is an error, the basal has not been obtained; the administrator therefore has to go back to the starting point and work backward until there are eight correct consecutive responses. Occasionally—especially with a young child—the administrator will not be able to work backward far enough to establish a basal, because the child will literally run out of test plates before the necessary eight correct consecutive responses can be obtained. In such a case, plate number one will be used as the basal.

To find the ceiling, testing continues forward from the point of the child's first error until the child makes six errors in eight consecutive plates. To repeat, the basal is the lowest of eight consecutive correct answers, and the ceiling is the highest item when there have been six errors out of eight consecutive responses.

Once the child's basal and ceiling have been determined, the test administrator can score the Peabody. At the top of page 3 inside of Score Sheet Form A is a space for recording the ceiling. When that has been done, the number of errors the child made between the ceiling and the basal are counted and recorded; this is subtracted from the ceiling number to obtain a raw score. This raw score is then recorded on the front of the scoring form in the space provided. Although there are also spaces for recording a computation of the child's I.Q., it is strongly urged that this not be done. The Peabody is an excellent test of language ability for children of a certain age, but it is not an I.Q. test, since it does not test a sufficient sample of cognitive or intellectual skills to be a valid test of I.Q.

Instead, test administrators are urged to turn to the table on page 12 of the Peabody manual which permits extrapolation of mental ages from raw scores. There are separate columns for scores. The administrator should note that there are also separate columns for computing mental age for Forms A and B, and should ensure that he or she is looking at the correct column. When the mental age has been found, it should be recorded on the front of the test form in the space provided.

INTERPRETING LANGUAGE TEST RESULTS

The next question is how to interpret the scores obtained on the REEL and Peabody. The Receptive and Expressive Language Ages obtained on the REEL and the Mental Age on the Peabody should be compared to the child's chronological age. The difference between them should be checked against Table 7–6, which will indicate whether the delay is a cause for concern, or an indication of the need for immediate referral.

For example, Table 7–6 shows that from birth to 12 months of age, a delay of two to three months is a cause for "concern." A delay of more than three months

(in comparison to the child's chronological age) indicates that referral and intervention are required. As the child gets older the amount of delay that can be considered a cause for "concern" rather than indication of "referral" gets larger. This becomes clear when one realizes that a three-month delay in a 12-month-old infant is a larger proportion of developmental life than a three-month delay in a five-year-old.

INTERVENTION AND REFERRAL

Table 7–7 indicates what should be done for specific causes of a speech and language delay. Children who demonstrate any amount of delay should have their hearing tested. This is best done by an audiologist. If none is available in the community, a speech pathologist experienced in such testing can be utilized. If neither of these resources is available, the physician should refer the child to the nearest hospital with an audiologist, or to an otolaryngologist who has an audiologist on the staff.

If hearing is intact and the language delay is in the column labeled "concern" (Table 7–6), and—even more important—if the delay appears to result from a depressed environment, the physician could try using some resource literature to increase the family's stimulation of the child. One book which the physician can use is titled *Teach Your Child to Talk*, a full reference for which appears in the Bibliography at the end of this chapter. This book presents normal speech and language development by age levels, offers questions to help the physician assist the parents in determining if speech and language are developing normally, and suggests activities in the home to stimu-

TABLE 7–6 Significance of Receptive or Expressive Language Delays

Age	Concern	Refer
0–12 months	2–3 months delay	More than 3 months delay
13–24 months	3–4 months delay	More than 4 months delay
25–36 months	4–5 months delay	More than 5 months delay
37–48 months	5–6 months delay	More than 6 months delay
49–60 months	6–9 months delay	More than 9 months delay

TABLE 7-7 Treating a Speaking Delay

Problem	What to Do	Where to Refer
1. Environmental		
a. Low socioeconomic level	a. Increase stimulation	a. Resource literature, Head Start, preschool
b. Family pressure	b. Decrease pressure	b. Counseling for family
c. Nonverbal family	c. Increase stimulation	c. Resource literature, Head Start, preschool
d. Bilingual home	d. Simplify language input	d. Refer to speech therapist and use of resource literature
2. Emotional		
a. Depressed mother	a. Increase stimulation	a. Refer for counseling, Head Start, preschool
b. Seriously disturbed parent	b. Stabilize emotional environment	b. Refer for psychotherapy
c. Seriously disturbed child	c. Improve emotional state of child	c. Refer for psychotherapy
3. Hearing Problems		
a. Congenital	a. Monitor and treat	a. Refer to audiologist and ENT specialist
b. Acquired	b. Monitor and treat	b. Refer to audiologist and ENT specialist
4. Developmental Delay		
a. Low average	a. Increase stimulation	a. Resource literature, preschool speech pathologist
b. Slow development	b. Increase stimulation	b. Resource literature, preschool speech pathologist
c. Mental retardation	c. Maximize potential	c. Special programs, community center, special Head Starts, speech pathologists, and resource literature
5. Birth Defects		
a. Cleft palate	a. Monitor and treat	a. Refer to cleft palate clinic
b. Down Syndrome	b. Monitor and treat	b. Refer to speech pathologist, birth defects clinic, special preschools, monitor for hearing loss
6. Brain Damage		
a. Neuromuscular damage	a. Overcome feeding problems and enhance speech development	a. Refer to occupational therapist, nutritionist, or speech pathologist
b. Sensorimotor	b. Overcome feeding problems and enhance speech development	b. Refer to occupational therapist, nutritionist, or speech therapist
c. Cerebral palsy	c. Maximize physical and cognitive development, enhance speech and language development	c. Refer to cerebral palsy centers with physical therapist, occupational therapist, and speech therapist
d. Perceptual problems	d. Overcome speech and language delays	d. Refer to speech pathologist and preschools

late speech and language development. For example, from four to six months of age, a child should make voice sounds while playing alone. Suggestions to help to stimulate a child's interest and vocalization include putting mobiles above the crib, or making a cradle gym of items at home, such as spoons and thread spools.

The physician should select one or two stimulation activities appropriate for the language age the child is showing and should discuss doing these activities with the family. This way the family will develop a feeling of accomplishment, and the child will benefit from focus on the stimulation. In addition, the child can be referred to a preschool or Head Start program.

This stimulation approach should be used for two months, and then the child should be reevaluated with the REEL or Peabody. If upon re-testing the delay remains at the "concern" level, the stimulation program should be continued. If the delay in language falls further below the chronological age to the "refer" level, then the child should be referred to a speech pathologist.

If the minimal delay is due to depression in one of the parents, sometimes the physician can directly counsel the parent. Here, too, the child might also be referred to a preschool or Head Start program for additional stimulation. However, if the depression is more serious, the parent should be referred for counseling. If the child is showing by history or action any emotional problems, the family should be referred for professional help in this area even before they are referred to a speech pathologist.

For the child who is mentally retarded, speech and language will usually be one of the more delayed areas. Such a child should be referred to a speech pathologist and put into a special school setting as soon as the problem is noted. This can help maximize the child's development.

Birth defects are generally identified very early. For this reason, children with birth defects can be put into the appropriate referral channels immediately. This can include special clinics dealing with specific problems. In addition, special schooling will be required and extra speech and language stimulation will probably be needed. The sooner the child can be put into programs specializing in developmental problems, the more optimal the programming that can be instituted.

Brain damage referral procedures vary with the problems the child presents. For early feeding problems, the most immediate need is to have the family seen by someone who can help with oral-motor stimulation; this can be an occupational therapist, nutritionist, or speech pathologist. If the damage encompasses the overall motor system, resulting in cerebral palsy, then the family should be referred to centers which have a staff trained in dealing with multiple problems.

If, however, the problems are more specifically related to language processing, then the speech pathologist should be the referral source. The speech pathologist can help the child develop speech and language skills, and can help prevent later school learning problems.

REFERRAL PROCEDURES

Table 7–8 provides a form which the physician can use for consultations on speech and language problems. When referring, the physician should send the following information: the amount of delay observed; other developmental lags; significant information from the history and medical examination; results of any developmental and speech and language testing; observational information on reception, association, and expression; and informed speculation about the type of problem that the child may have.

In turn, the physician should request information about whether or not there are significant speech and language problems. If so, to what degree? What type of problem is it? What seem to be the

---

TABLE 7–8   Consult Request for Speech and Language Referral

Information to Send
1. Amount of delay observed in speech and language
2. Other developmental lags observed
3. Significant problem areas from developmental history
4. Type of problem as the physician sees it

Information to Request
1. Are there significant speech and language delays? To what extent?
2. What kind of problem(s)?
3. Cause(s)?
4. Recommendation(s)?
5. Long-term prognosis?

---

causes? What is the recommended intervention approach? And what is the tentative long-term prognosis?

Sometimes the physician delays a referral in order to save the parents unnecessary concern. Probably a better approach is to share with the parents information about a consultation. The parents should understand that the referral is an effort to find out *if* this is a problem, and if so, whether intervention is required. The physician who is concerned should refer when the delay indicates that this is appropriate.

Referral sources in each community can be found among universities that have a department of communication disorders, hospitals that have a department of speech therapy, private clinics, rehabilitation centers, or private therapists. The physician should establish a community resource list so that such resources will be available when referral is needed.

ARTICULATION

It is difficult to assess whether or not a child is saying all the appropriate sounds. Because it requires specific training and practice, articulation training will not be covered in this chapter. However, since it is frequently important to assess articulation, it is recommended that someone in each physician's office learn to administer an articulation test.

(For a training tape and materials needed to conduct one such test, the Denver Articulation Screening Examination, contact: LADOCA Publishing Foundation, East 51st Avenue at Lincoln Street, Denver, Colorado 80216. Telephone 303-629-6379.)

SUMMARY

This chapter has covered many points: a conceptual model of language functioning; milestones of speech and language development; causes of speech and language problems; clinical observation of speech and language; methods of intervention; and procedures for referral.

One of the most important things for the physician to keep in mind is that any system in the child that shows damage or delay may affect speech and language development. Speech and language, to be most intact, require that every other system be intact, for speech is the last-developed species-specific trait of the human being. Speech development is sensitive to interruptions in any other system, including the environmental, emotional, cognitive, neurological, and physiological structure. Any problem in any of these areas signals that speech and language may not develop normally.

The final point in this chapter is the same as the first point: remember that talking is normal while not talking— ain't.

APPENDIX A

Clinical Guide for Use of the REEL

RECEPTIVE LANGUAGE	**EXPRESSIVE LANGUAGE**

Zero to One Month

____R1. What does (s)he do when (s)he hears a loud, sudden noise?

____R2. If (s)he is in his/her chair or crib and you come toward him/her while talking to him/her—or if the dog comes into the room and barks—what does (s)he do?

____R3. If (s)he is fussy and you're busy, can (s)he be quieted by your talking? Or do you need to pick him/her up?

____E1. Does (s)he cry a lot?

____E2. Does (s)he make sounds other than crying?

____E3. Are the sounds (s)he makes mostly open mouth sounds? For instance, does (s)he not really say words, but just make sounds with his/her mouth open like "aah" or "eee?"

One to Two Months

____R4. If you're holding him/her, and there are other people around besides you who are talking, does (s)he notice them or pay attention to them?

____R5. If (s)he is sitting or lying in the crib and you talk to him/her, what is his/her response? How does (s)he show his/her response?

____R6. If you are talking to him/her, does (s)he look at you and smile?

____E4. Does (s)he have a special cry for hunger?

____E5. When (s)he's just making sounds, like cooing or babbling, does (s)he sometimes repeat the same syllable like "duh-duh-duh" or "dee-dee-dee?"

____E6. Does (s)he show in any particular way that (s)he's happy? Does (s)he make some particular sounds when (s)he's feeling good?

Two to Three Months

____R7. When you're talking to him/her, where does (s)he look?

____R8. If (s)he's sitting in a room where there are people talking, does (s)he regularly look and look at them?

____R9. When someone is talking, does (s)he ever look at their lips and mouth?

____E7. When (s)he hears music or television, or if you're talking to him/her, does (s)he occasionally respond to this by making sounds?

____E8. When you play with him/her, does (s)he laugh or make other sounds to show you that (s)he's having fun and feels good?

____E9. Does (s)he often make two or more different syllables, such as "a-da," "e-be," or "e-ba?"

RECEPTIVE LANGUAGE	EXPRESSIVE LANGUAGE

Three to Four Months

____R10. If (s)he's sitting in a chair or lying on the floor and (s)he hears someone talking, does (s)he turn his/her head toward that person?

____R11. Does (s)he seem to look around to try and find the person who is speaking?

____R12. If you are angry and yelling at one of the children or at the dog, does (s)he become frightened or disturbed? How does (s)he show this?

____E10. Does (s)he often laugh when (s)he's playing with toys or things?

____E11. When (s)he's playing—especially when (s)he's playing by herself/himself—does (s)he, regularly take a sound and repeat it over and over again? Sounds like "ba-ba-ba-ba-ba?"

____E12. Will (s)he often make sounds like "p-p-p" or "m-m-m" or "b-b-b" with his/her lips?

Four to Five Months

____R13. Can (s)he look around and pretty regularly locate who is talking?

____R14. Does (s)he respond to his/her own name?

____R15. If (s)he's crying and you talk to him/her, is that enough to comfort him/her? Or do you need to pick him/her up?

____E13. Will (s)he make sounds now like "oh" or "ooh?"

____E14. Will (s)he let you know that (s)he's angry or not too happy by making sounds other than crying?

____E15. When (s)he's making his/her babbling sounds and you talk to him/her, will (s)he usually stop babbling? Even though (s)he may continue making sounds for a little while, will (s)he usually stop babbling and listen to you?

Five to Six Months

____R16. Can (s)he tell the difference between: (1) when you are a little irritated, (2) when you're really angry, and (3) when you're feeling kind of loving? How does (s)he show that (s)he knows the difference in the tones of your voice?

____R17. Does (s)he recognize words like "daddy," "bye-bye," "ma-ma?" How does (s)he show that?

____R18. Does (s)he stop what (s)he's doing at least half the time when you say "no?"

____E16. Does (s)he ever babble to you on his/her own—not just in response to your talking to him/her?

____E17. Will (s)he occasionally make four or more different sounds in a row, like "ah-bee-dah-boo?"

____E18. Will (s)he play at making sounds and noises? When (s)he's alone or with others, does (s)he just seem to enjoy making sounds?

RECEPTIVE LANGUAGE	EXPRESSIVE LANGUAGE

Six to Seven Months

R19. If you're talking and you refer to "Daddy" or "Grandma," or if you say the name of your baby's brother or sister, will (s)he look around or show in some way that (s)he recognizes the name?

E19. Is (s)he beginning to use two different sounds when (s)he babbles, rather than using a string of the same sounds? I mean, is (s)he now making more sounds like "buh-duh" or "muh-duh" rather than "buh-buh-buh."

R20. If you look at him/her and say, "come" or "up," will (s)he raise his/her arms? Or if you say "bye-bye," will (s)he wave?

E20. When you call him/her by name, does (s)he make some sound at least half the time?

R21. If (s)he hears music on the radio, record player, or TV, or if you play a musical toy, does (s)he seem to listen to it?

E21. Does (s)he use any sounds that almost seem to mean words to him/her? For example, does (s)he use a made-up word for a favorite toy, a pet, or some food (s)he likes?

Seven to Eight Months

_____R22. If your child is sitting in a room while you talk with your spouse or a friend, does (s)he often seem to really listen to the whole conversation?

_____E22. Does (s)he sometimes make a long string of sounds, almost like a sentence even though there aren't any real words yet?

_____R23. Does (s)he regularly stop what (s)he's doing when you call his/her name?

_____E23. Does (s)he play any games like "patty-cake" or "peek-a-boo?"

_____R24. Does (s)he seem to recognize names of everyday things around the house when you name them, things like ball or dog? How does (s)he show that (s)he recognizes them?

_____E24. If (s)he hears some song or music that (s)he likes, will (s)he make noises as if (s)he were singing along with it?

Eight to Nine Months

_____R25. Does (s)he seem to understand some simple requests from you, such as, "Look here," or "Let me see it?" How does (s)he show that?

_____E25. Does (s)he use any gestures to let you know what she means, such as shaking his/her head for "no?"

_____R26. Does (s)he regularly stop what (s)he's doing when you say "no?" You notice that *before,* I asked if (s)he stopped what (s)he's doing when you say "no" at least *half* the time. Now I'm asking if (s)he *regularly* stops what (s)he's doing when you say "no."

_____E26. Will (s)he often imitate sounds and the same *number* of sounds that you make when talking with her? For example, if you say, "ba-ba," will (s)he say "ba-ba" back?

_____R27. Can (s)he sit and look at pictures for a full minute if you also sit and look at them and name them for him/her?

_____E27. Does (s)he make more sounds like "gah," "bah," or "dah" (not just the open mouth sounds like "ooh" and "o") than (s)he did when (s)he was six months of age?

RECEPTIVE LANGUAGE	EXPRESSIVE LANGUAGE

Nine to Ten Months

____R28. Does (s)he seem to enjoy listening to new words? How does (s)he show that?

____E28. Is (s)he beginning to use any words? Does (s)he use them often? For example, does (s)he often say, "da-da," "ma-ma," "bye-bye," or the name of a pet or a toy?

____R29. If you're talking to him/her, will (s)he pay attention? Or if you're talking to him/her and something happens outside or a truck goes by, does that take his/her attention?

____E29. Is (s)he using any exclamations (like "Oh!" for a warning that there is danger, or "eee," meaning that something is nice)?

____R30. Will (s)he *often* give toys or other things (s)he has to you when you say, "Give it to me?" Notice that I am saying *often*.

____E30. Will (s)he often try to "talk" to you in what we would call jargon sentences? Does it sound like (s)he's really talking to you, even though there are no real words coming through?

Ten to Eleven Months

____R31. Will (s)he sometimes follow simple commands like, "Put that down?"

____E31. When (s)he's playing alone, does (s)he usually make different strings of sounds?

____R32. Does (s)he seem to understand simple questions like, "Where is the ball?" How does (s)he show it?

____E32. Will (s)he come up to you and try to get you to play "patty-cake" or "peek-a-boo" because (s)he wants to—not just in response to you?

____R33. Will (s)he respond to music by moving his/her body or hands, not necessarily keeping good rhythm, but kind of moving to the music?

____E33. Will (s)he sometimes try to imitate new words that you are saying to him/her?

Eleven to Twelve Months

____R34. Does (s)he make some appropriate gestures when you ask him/her to, like "Give me your hand," or "Close your eyes," or "Hold up your foot?"

____E34. Do you think (s)he uses three or more words pretty consistently?

____R35. Generally, does (s)he seem really interested and does (s)he respond when you talk to him/her for long periods of time?

____E35. Does (s)he talk to his/her toys and to people all day long, using long strings of sounds?

____R36. Will (s)he give you verbal responses when you ask him/her to? For instance, when you ask him/her to say "bye-bye," will (s)he say "bye-bye?"

____E36. Does (s)he often respond to songs or rhymes that (s)he hears by vocalizing back?

RECEPTIVE LANGUAGE	EXPRESSIVE LANGUAGE

Twelve to Fourteen Months

____R37. Does (s)he seem to understand some new words each week? (Or maybe it isn't coming in that fast yet?)

____R38. Does (s)he seem to understand your feelings or the feelings of most people around him/her? For example, if your husband comes home tired and a little bit edgy, does (s)he show that (s)he understands the difference from when your husband comes home untired and ready to play? How does (s)he show that (s)he understands the difference?

____R39. Can (s)he sit and look at pictures that you are naming for up to two minutes at a time?

____E37. Does (s)he use five or more true words pretty consistently?

____E38. Does (s)he try to get things (s)he wants by using his/her voice along with pointing or gesturing? (S)he may not necessarily say the words, but may say some "ah," "e," or "um" sounds while pointing.

____E39. Are some *true* words now coming through when (s)he's trying to talk with long strings of sounds?

Fourteen to Sixteen Months

____R40. Can (s)he bring something from another room if you ask him/her to? What sort of things will (s)he bring?

____R41. Can (s)he recognize some everyday things or pictures of them if you name them and you ask him/her to point to them? What things could (s)he recognize?

____R42. Could (s)he recognize very easily parts of his/her own body, such as eyes, hair, mouth, ears, and hands?

____E40. Does (s)he use seven or more true words pretty consistently?

____E41. Is (s)he using sounds like "ta," "da," "wa," "mm," or "ha," like sounds in the words we use?

____E42. When (s)he's trying to communicate with you, does (s)he use some true words along with the gestures? There may be a lot of the sounds still, but does (s)he use some true words?

Sixteen to Eighteen Months

____R43. Can (s)he understand and carry out two instructions in a row? For example, can (s)he pick up a ball and put it in a box, or go get his/her shoes and put them in the closet?

____R44. Can (s)he associate new words by connecting them to other things

____E43. Is (s)he beginning to use words rather than pointing to let you know what (s)he wants or needs? Is (s)he beginning to be able to name the things that (s)he wants, and to use enough words that you can tell what (s)he wants?

____E44. Is (s)he beginning to repeat words (s)he has heard when you talk?

RECEPTIVE LANGUAGE

that (s)he knows? For instance, if
(s)he understands that (s)he eats
toast, will (s)he understand that
toast and crackers and bread are all
foods that you eat? If (s)he knows
shoes and (s)he sees boots, can (s)he
realize that boots and shoes and
coats are all things you wear?
_____R45. If there were four things in
front of him/her—a ball, a shoe,
a sock, and a toy—and you asked
for two of those things, could
(s)he select them and give them
to you?

EXPRESSIVE LANGUAGE

_____E45. Do you think (s)he's showing
a continual, gradual increase in the
words that (s)he can and does use?

Eighteen to Twenty Months

_____R46. If you showed him/her some
pictures, could (s)he point to
hair, nose, mouth, or shoes?
Before, I asked if (s)he could
point to them on himself/herself.
Now, it's a little bit more
difficult: can (s)he point to
them in a picture?
_____R47. Does (s)he do things that you
ask him/her to do like "Sit down,"
"Stand up," "Come here," or
"Stop that?"
_____R48. Does (s)he understand the
difference between "Give it to
me," "Give it to her," or "Give
it to him?" Would (s)he understand
and do it correctly?

_____E46. Does (s)he imitate some two
or three word sentences that (s)he
hears you or others make?

_____E47. Does (s)he imitate any sounds
that (s)he hears around him/her
when (s)he's playing, like motor
sounds, or animal sounds?
_____E48. Do you think (s)he uses
at least 10 to 20 words when (s)he
talks?

Twenty to Twenty-Two Months

_____R49. Can (s)he do two or three very
simple but related things if you
gave him/her directions to do it?
For instance, could (s)he (1) get the
toy, pick it up, and bring it
to you? Or (2) pick up the ball,
put it in the closet, and close the
door?
_____R50. Does (s)he seem to recognize
new words almost every day, or is
it not coming in that fast yet?
_____R51. Does (s)he seem to recognize
almost all everyday objects or

_____E49. Is (s)he beginning to combine
words into several sentences, like
"Go bye-bye" or "Daddy come?"

_____E50. Does (s)he speak and use more
new words each week? Is it coming
in that fast?
_____E51. Does (s)he try to tell you about
what (s)he's done? Let's say

RECEPTIVE LANGUAGE	EXPRESSIVE LANGUAGE

pictures of everyday objects if you name them?

(s)he's been outside playing and wants to come in and tell you "Big doggy," or "Somebody ran fast." Does (s)he try and tell you even if it's sometimes true words mixed with a string of sounds that aren't quite true words?

Twenty-Two to Twenty-Four Months

____R52. Out of five things in front of him/her—for instance a comb, spoon, cup, dog, and sock—could (s)he take one and give that to you when you ask him/her to?

____E52. Does (s)he occasionally use three-word sentences, like "There it is," "Play with blocks," "We go now," or "No more cookie?"

____R53. Does (s)he seem to listen to the meaning and the reason of what you're saying—not just the words or the sound? For instance, if you say, "Don't put your hand there; it's hot," will (s)he realize what that means and keep his/her hand away?

____E53. Does (s)he refer to himself by using his/her own name?

____R54. Does (s)he seem to understand pretty grownup sentences? If you said, "When we get to the store, I'll buy you an ice cream cone," would (s)he remember that? How would (s)he show you that (s)he understood that?

____E54. Does (s)he use some pronouns like I, me, or you? Even though (s)he is sometimes making mistakes, is (s)he trying to use them?

Twenty-Four to Twenty-Seven Months

____R55. Does (s)he understand words about things you do? For instance, if you were looking at pictures of eating, running, walking, and sleeping, and you asked, "Which one is sleeping?" or "Which one is walking?" could (s)he point to the right picture?

____E55. Does (s)he usually use a two- or three-word sentence? Earlier I was asking if (s)he's *beginning* to use two- to three-word sentences; now I'm asking if (s)he *usually* uses two- or three-word sentences.

____R56. Can (s)he point to smaller parts of the body such as the chin, elbow, eyebrow, ankle, and so on?

____E56. Does (s)he *often* use pronouns like I, you, he, it, or me?

____R57. Does (s)he understand family names like Baby, Grandma, Mama? How does (s)he show that?

____E57. Does (s)he ask for some things that (s)he wants, like help to wash his/her hands or to go to the bathroom?

Twenty-Seven to Thirty Months

____R58. Does (s)he understand questions like, "What do you eat with?" "What do you wear?" Can (s)he answer appropriately?

____E58. Can (s)he name at least one color correctly?

RECEPTIVE LANGUAGE

___R59. Does (s)he understand size yet? For example, can (s)he pick out the little ball from the big ball?

___R60. Can (s)he recognize names and pictures of most everyday objects? Before, I asked for *almost* all. Now we're going for *most* objects.

Thirty to Thirty-Three Months

___R61. Does (s)he seem to understand most words about the things you do, like running, walking, eating, sleeping, crying, washing? How does (s)he demonstrate that (s)he understands those words?

___R62. Does (s)he seem to understand really long and involved sentences, almost to the point where you don't have to simplify much for his/her age anymore?

___R63. Does (s)he seem to understand words that are used to describe things? For example, does (s)he understand words like "dirty," or "broken?" Would (s)he pick out or throw away a "dirty dish" or a "broken toy" if you asked him/her to?

Thirty-Three to Thirty-Six Months

___R64. Does (s)he seem to want to know why or how things work—not just because it *is* or because it *happens* that way? What does (s)he do to let you know that (s)he wants to know this?

___R65. Can (s)he do three simple things that you tell him/her to do at one time, such as, "Come inside, wash your hands and sit at the table?" Or "Come inside, put your toys away, and get ready to go to bed?"

___R66. Does (s)he understand prepositions, things like on, under, in front of, or behind? How does (s)he show that (s)he understands these?

EXPRESSIVE LANGUAGE

___E59. Does (s)he refer to himself/herself by using a pronoun instead of his/her own name? For example, does (s)he say, "I want a cookie," instead of "(Child's name) wants a cookie?"

___E60. Can (s)he repeat two or more numbers correctly? For example, if you ask him/her to say "three–two," can (s)he say both numbers back?

___E61. Can (s)he tell if (s)he's a boy or a girl if you ask him/her?

___E62. If (s)he's drawing and you ask what (s)he's drawing, will (s)he name it and tell you about it?

___E63. Can (s)he say both his/her first and last name (his/her full name) when you ask him/her to?

___E64. Earlier I sked if (s)he tries to tell you what (s)he's been doing. Now I'm going to ask if (s)he *regularly* tells you what (s)he's been doing or what happened when (s)he was out playing or visiting a friend.

___E65. If (s)he's telling stories about what is going on in a picture, can (s)he use words to describe action, such as, "They are going swimming," "They are going to sleep," or "They were sleeping (or eating or washing)?"

___E66. Is (s)he able to use plurals? For instance, does (s)he refer to two shoes as shoes, to more than one dog as doggies, and so on?

BIBLIOGRAPHY

Bang, T. E. *Language and learning disorders of the pre-academic child.* New York: Appleton-Century-Crofts, 1968.

Bzoch, K. R., and League, R. *Receptive-expressive emergent language scale.* Baltimore: University Park Press, n.d.

Carrow, M. A. Clinical model of human communication. In M.S. Preston (Ed.), Psycholinguistics and the evaluation of language function. *Pediatric Clinics of North America,* 1973, *20,* 79–88.

Dunn, L. M. *Peabody picture vocabulary test.* Circle Pines, Minn: American Guidance, 1965.

Morley, M. E. *The development and disorders of speech in childhood* (3rd ed.). Baltimore: Williams and Wilkins, 1972.

Osgood, C. E., and Miron, M. S. *Approaches to the study of aphasia.* Urbana: University of Illinois Press, 1963.

Pushaw, D. R. *Teach your child to talk.* Fairfield, N.J.: Cebco/Standard, 1976.

Rutter, M., and Martin, J. A. M. *The child with delayed speech.* Philadelphia: J. B. Lippincott, 1972.

Wood, N. E. *Verbal learning: Part I—Language acquisition.* San Rafael: University of California, 1969.

Wepman, J. M., Jones, L. V., and Van Pelt, D. Studies in aphasia: Backgrounds and theoretical formulations. *Journal of Speech and Hearing Disorders,* 1960, *29,* 323–332.

Chapter 8

Goal

To develop skills in the assessment and diagnosis of children with neurological and neuromotor problems.

Objectives

At the end of this chapter, the physician should be able to:

- identify a history that is a risk factor in considering a neurological or neuromotor problem;
- identify significant neurological and neuromotor symptoms;
- determine when to refer a child for neuromotor and neurological problems.

NEUROLOGICAL EVALUATION

By

LAWRENCE H. BERNSTEIN, M.D.

I. Introduction

The goal of this chapter is to help the physician recognize when neurological disease is responsible for a developmental delay and know what should be done about it.

II. The Medical History and Physical Examination

A. The physician should explore the history by using the Parent Questionnaire (Appendix A in Chapter 4) and the History of the Present Illness Form (Appendix C in Chapter 4).

B. Next, the physician should identify aspects of the Medical Examination which have potential neurological implications, by using Appendix D of Chapter 4.

C. Items in the Parent Questionnaire, the History of the Present Illness, and the Medical Examination form which have possible neurological implications have been preceded with an "N."

III. The Neuromotor Developmental Examination

A. A simple and brief developmental examination for use with children 24 months of age or less is the Milani Comparetti Neuromotor Developmental Examination.

B. When completed, the Milani Comparetti developmental chart provides a profile of the infant's motor function in relationship to the expected ages of appearance and disappearance of primitive and developmental reflexes.

C. The four major components of the evaluation are righting reactions, parachute reactions, tilting reactions, and primitive reflexes.

IV. The Neurological Examination

A. After evaluating a child for neuromotor development, the physician should conduct a thorough neurological examination.

B. Appendix B of this chapter is a Neurological Examination Checklist for use during the examination.

V. Intracranial Lesions

A. One intracranial lesion is microcephaly; this includes primary (or congenital) microcephaly, and secondary microcephaly.

B. Primary microcephaly usually reflects problems arising early in pregnancy and is immediately evident at birth; possible causes include intrauterine insults such as congenital infections, X-ray procedures during the first trimester, and familial, inherited forms.

C. Secondary microcephaly may reflect insults to the brain late in pregnancy, at the time of delivery, or after delivery; affected children have small, but normally-shaped heads.

D. A rare cause of microcephaly is craniosynostosis of all sutures; single suture closure does not cause microcephaly.

E. Another type of lesion is intracranial bleeding caused by birth trauma or by postnatal causes such as falls or blows to the head.

F. A third type of intracranial process is hydrocephalus resulting

from a blockage in the flow of spinal fluid, a blockage in the resorption of spinal fluid, or excessive production of spinal fluid.
   G. Whenever an intracranial lesion is suspected, the child should be referred to a neurologist for an extensive evaluation.
VI. Cerebral Palsy
   A. Cerebral palsy is often secondary to a static intracranial neurological impairment, and is commonly associated with prematurity, intracranial hemorrhage, hypoxia, and kernicterus.
   B. Signs of an intracranial lesion may—or may not—be found with cerebral palsy; there will probably be delays in motor development or persistence of primary motor patterns upon evaluation with the Milani Comparetti, and the more traditional neurologic signs may be seen by a year and one-half of age.
   C. Although some children with cerebral palsy also manifest intellectual impairment, many are intellectually normal.
   D. Children with cerebral palsy should be referred to physical or occupational theraptists to teach or facilitate functional development of normal movement patterns, to prevent the development of contractures and deformities, and to assist the parents in dealing with the child.
   E. The neurodevelopmental treatment approach of the Bobaths involves the inhibition of patterns of abnormal reflex activity and facilitation of normal motor patterns.
VII. Minor Motor Seizures
   A. Minor motor seizures are an infrequent cause of delays, especially of delays in intellectual development.
   B. Symptoms include poor attention span, decreased comprehension, staring spells, inappropriate pauses in speech, unusual facial movements, repetitive movements, and sudden alterations in body posture or tone; signs include cerebral dysgenesis and skin lesions.
   C. A child suspected of minor motor seizure disorders should be referred to a child neurologist for an evaluation.
VIII. Peripheral Neuropathy
   A. Peripheral neuropathy may be due to a variety of conditions, including toxic metabolic disease, Guillain-Barre, Werdnig-Hoffman infantile muscular atrophy, and heredito-familial diseases or degenerative disorders.
   B. Symptoms and signs will depend upon which nerves are involved; mental status is generally intact.
   C. A child with peripheral neuropathy should be referred to a neurologist.
IX. Muscle Diseases
   A. Muscle diseases, although quite rare, should be kept in mind when evaluating a child who seems slow in motor development or who manifests signs of hypotonia.
   B. Generally, muscle diseases start gradually after infancy, and often there is a positive family history.
   C. The differential diagnosis of muscle disease would be muscular dystrophy, myasthenia gravis, dermatomyositis, periodic paralysis, and endocrine disorders.
   D. Any child suspected of a muscle disease should be referred to the nearest muscle disease clinic or neurologist.
X. Degenerative Disorders
   A. Although degenerative disorders are extremely rare, they are generally not treatable; it is important they be identified for family counseling purposes.
   B. Symptoms and signs will depend upon the type of degenerative disorder, the etiology, and the site of the lesion; any child suspected of such disorder should be referred to a neurologist.
XI. Summary

INTRODUCTION

When a developmental delay is not caused by an orthopedic, metabolic, or endocrine abnormality, in many cases an abnormality of the nervous system is implied. Because of this, it is important for the physician in his or her decision-making process to: discriminate between a static encephalopathy and a progressive central nervous system lesion; discern whether the disability is permanent, whether it is remediable, or whether it is self-correcting; and identify when a potentially remediable condition is causing the developmental delay. The goal of this chapter is to help the physician recognize when neurological disease is responsible for a developmental delay and what should be done about it.

To enable the primary care physician to identify the disorders referred to above and to make appropriate referrals, the first goal of this lesson is to teach the physician to identify intracranial lesions, cerebral palsy, minor motor seizures, peripheral neuropathy, muscle disease, and degenerative disorders. The second major objective is to teach the physician what to do if a child having any of these disorders is encountered.

THE MEDICAL HISTORY AND PHYSICAL EXAMINATION

Many of the questions which the physician will ask to establish the presence or absence of disease of the nervous system are outlined in the printed Parent Questionnaire (Appendix A in Chapter 4), and the History of the Present Illness form (Appendix C in Chapter 4). The physician should ordinarily begin with the presenting complaint, which may be a delay or a regression in the child's motor, intellectual, or social-emotional development. After exploring this in some detail to learn the onset of the disorder and how it has progressed, the physician should look into the family history for historical risk factors. To assist in identification of items which may be of neurological significance, the questions that have potential neurological implications have been preceded with an "N" in these appendices.

The second step in identifying significant neurological disorders is to identify aspects of the medical examination which have potential neurological implications. (The physical findings of syndromes that have neurological implications are discussed in Chapter 10.) As in the case of the history, the items have potential neurological significance are preceded with an "N" in Appendix D of Chapter 4.

THE NEUROMOTOR DEVELOPMENTAL EXAMINATION

The third step is to conduct careful developmental and neurological examinations of the integrity of the central nervous system. The two differ in aims and techniques. Since the infant and preschool-age child's neurological system is still developing, there is a need to determine the age-appropriateness of the child's motor, language, and emotional development, as well as the localizing signs of the more traditional neurological examination. As Towen has pointed out, *both* the developmental and the neurological evaluations serve important needs; that is, they are complimentary, and one cannot replace the other.

A simple, brief, and useful developmental examination which can be used in developmental diagnosis is the Milani Comparetti Neuromotor Developmental Examination. This examination is designed for use with children who are 24 months of age or less. It provides a standardized way of examining a child's primitive and developmental reflexes by stressing the evaluation of primary motor patterns* along the developmental continuum. The procedures provide an opportunity for direct visual evaluation of age-related, spontaneous motor patterns (such as postural control of the head or trunk, the protective or parachute reactions, etc.) evoked as a result of the body's

---

*Comparetti more recently no longer talks of "primitive reflexes;" rather, he now calls them "primary motor patterns." He writes: "Within the developmental perspective the fact that a certain motor behavior can be evoked by a stimulus does not reduce it to a reflex [i.e., according to the model of the reflex arch]..."

response to gravity (i.e., anti-gravity control of the body axis). The Milani Comparetti developmental chart, when completed, provides a profile of the infant's motor function in relationship to the expected ages of appearance and disappearance. Thus, the examination is not only suited for the evaluation of a child who is suspected of manifesting a developmental deviation, but can also be used to monitor the development of infants as a part of periodic health visits. When performing the examination, one looks for asymmetry, delayed onset of primitive reflexes, or abnormal persistence of primitive reflexes. There are four major components of the Milani Comparetti evaluation, which are as follows:

a. The first is righting reactions, which are important for achieving erect body posture; this includes head and body righting, as well as derotative righting. In head righting, the baby (when held in a vertical position and then tilted away from the vertical axis) will attempt to maintain the head in an upright position, with the eyes horizontal and the nose vertical. Body righting takes place when a 10-month-old child is put on his or her back; normally the child rolls over to prone and stands up. Derotive righting is an untwisting when rotation is applied to the long axis of the body. For instance, if the head is rotated, lower segments will tend to follow the turning of the head, and will therefore derotate the body.

b. The second type of evoked reactions—the parachute reactions—are reactions of the limbs to sudden replacement relative to gravity of the erect structure. For example, if a four-month-old child is suddenly moved downward toward a table in a vertical position, he or she will extend his or her upper limbs; if a seven-month-old child is moved suddenly forward, the upper limbs will move forward; if a nine-month-old is moved backward, he

or she will extend the arms backward.

c. The third kind of reactions are the tilting reactions. These are reactions to stimulating the body at an angular acceleration (or tilting) to prevent the tendency of falling. The central feature in these is curving of the spine.

d. The importance of the primary motor patterns of primitive reflexes (especially the tonic labyrinthine, asymmetric tonic neck, positive support, and less so the symmetric tonic neck reflex, Moro, and hand and foot grasp) lies in the fact that the baby utilizes them functionally in different ways, and that each functional use is a precise marker of the developmental process. For example, E. A. Gidoui wrote in *Developmental Medicine and Child Neurology* that the foot's plantar grasp response "...may be elicited even at two or three years of age, but when tested in this context—that is, when the child is standing—it must disappear before the child is able to stand with support [i.e., at about nine months]."

Excerpts from the Milani Comparetti Neuromotor Developmental Examination are reprinted with permission in Appendix A which accompanies this chapter. It is recommended that this be closely read by those wishing to learn how to conduct the examination.

THE NEUROLOGICAL EXAMINATION

The next step in evaluating a suspect child for neurological problems is to conduct a thorough neurological examination. The neurological examination of infants and small children differs significantly from that in adults and older children both because of the maturation of the nervous system and the inability or unwillingness of the child to cooperate in a formal examination. An initial observation of spontaneously-produced activity, posture, behaviors, and so forth, can often provide as much or more information than attempts to elicit the more formal responses. Examiners should also be prepared to modify the order and content of the examination to fit the child and the circumstances. A Neurological Exmaination Checklist is presented as Appendix B in this chapter. (Although certain aspects of the physical examination, such as head circumference, general alertness, and speech are important parts of the neurological examination, these have been omitted from the Checklist to avoid repetition.)

INTRACRANIAL LESIONS

There are several important neurological problems which the physician may encounter when evaluating children who are suspect on developmental screening; one such category includes intracranial lesions—and, of these, the first is microcephaly. It is important for the physician to know about and be aware of microcephaly because it is often an indication of neurological impairment.

There are two kinds of microcephaly—primary or congenital microcephaly, and secondary microcephaly. Primary microcephaly usually reflects problems arising early in pregnancy and is of such a degree as to be immediately evident at birth, when the cranial vault is relatively flat above the orbital ridges, the ears, and the occiput. Possible etiological factors include significant intrauterine insults such as congenital infections or X-ray procedures, particularly during the first trimester, and familial forms with varying patterns of inheritance. Microcephaly may also be inherited; genetic causes may suggest the need for karyotyping for trisomies or, in one rare autosymal dominant syndrome, an X-ray of the skull for intracranial calcifications. (These are discussed more fully in Chapter 10.) The diagnosis of microcephaly rests upon obtaining a measurement of the head circumference which is below the third percentile for the child's chronological age.

The next condition which must be considered is secondary microcephaly. Secondary or acquired microcephaly may reflect insults to the developing brain occurring late in pregnancy, at the time of delivery, or after delivery. Affected children have craniums that are normally contoured, but small. Microcephalic mentally retarded children are often relatively small; however, non-microcephalic children who are small should have normal brain growth, since the head growth is not dependent on the total body growth. In fact, in situations of intrauterine malnutrition, the last organ of the body to be impaired in growth is the brain. Thus, the child who fails to thrive for reason of gastrointestinal disorders—such as malabsorption—will usually continue to have a normal rate of cranial growth.

A rare cause of microcephaly which will be mentioned briefly is craniosynostosis of all sutures. Single suture closure does not cause microcephaly. It does produce a cosmetic deformity, but it generally does not lead to neurological or developmental problems.

Because of the possibility of the existence of microcephaly, it is important for the physician to measure the head circumference of all children who manifest delays in development. In the event that a child who manifests microcephaly is discovered, the physician must demonstrate that the child is functioning normally intellectually and otherwise, since microcephaly may reflect neurological impairment.

The second type of disorders of cerebral lesions which will be considered is intracranial bleeding. Sometimes such bleeding results from birth trauma, which in turn may be associated with precipitous deliveries, cephalopelvic disproportion, and breech deliveries. Postnatal causes of intracranial bleeding include falls or blows to the head (such as may be seen in accidents and cases of neglect or abuse). Such trauma may result in subdural hematomas, brain contusion, or subarachnoid hemorrhage.

A third type of intracranial lesion is hydrocephalus. This may result from: a blockage in the flow of spinal fluid that is seen in an Arnold-Chiari malformation; a blockage in the resorption of the cerebral spinal fluid following meningitis (subarachnoid hemorrhage); or the excessive production of spinal fluid from a choroid plexus papilloma. All of these conditions occupy space in the head. Therefore, they may produce pressure upon the existing brain tissue if the skull sutures have closed; or in the presence of unfused sutures, they may produce excessive enlargement of the head circumference. Thus, the signs and symptoms are to some extent age-related. More importantly, they relate to whether or not the cranial sutures had closed prior to the development of the space-taking lesion.

In general, symptoms are non-specific and may include headaches, nausea, vomiting, lethargy, irritability, and personality changes. An early sign that may be noticed is a change in the shape of the skull. This may be an excessive growth in the head circumference, so that the head circumference may change more than 50 percentile units within a relatively short period of time. Other signs may be the frontal bossing that is commonly seen with hydrocephalus, or bulging on one side of the head due to up-going subdural hematoma. For infants below two years of age, if an intracranial lesion is suspected, the physician is strongly urged to transilluminate the head. Transillumination may be positive when there is a very thin cortex secondary to hydrocephalus, or when there is fluid on top of the brain, as in hydranencephaly or subdural hematomas.

Other signs that might be seen when there is an intracranial process in the posterior fossa are a stiff neck and a head tilt. If the flow of spinal fluid is blocked, there will be an enlargement of the lateral ventricles; this in turn produces a stretching of the pyramidal fibers, especially those of the lower extremities. As a result, one may see poor coordination, hyperreflexia, ankle clonus, and an extensor plantar response (Babinski).

If trauma to the head is suspected, it is of paramount importance for the physician to thoroughly examine the retina to determine if there are any hemorrhages. During the neurological examination, there may be a variety of cranial nerve signs, including blurred vision, papilledema, enlargement of the blind spot, optic atrophy, abnormal eye movements, facial paralysis, and possibly cerebellar signs, including ataxia of the trunk, arms, and legs.

In addition, there may be corticospinal weakness of the wrist and finger extensors and of the hip and ankle flexors. Ankle clonus and upgoing toes should be checked for as well. If there is a focal space-occupying lesion, the physician may also find seizures, localized impaired function, and/or impairment in somatic growth.

In the event that a case of microcephaly is identified—even though it would generally be a static, non-progressive lesion—it is important for the physician to attempt to establish whether the microcephaly is primary or secondary. This may have implications in determining the etiology of the child's developmental problem, and may also have implications in counseling the parents regarding the probable course of the child's condition.

Whenever an intracranial space-taking lesion is suspected, it is very important that the primary care physician refer the child for a thorough evaluation. Most often such a referral will be to a neurologist for a very careful and more extensive evaluation. Though CAT scans can be helpful in identifying and localizing such lesions, the CAT scan is very expensive. Therefore, if the physician has sufficient concern to refer the child for a CAT scan, the child should first be referred to determine if, indeed, that kind of diagnostic evaluation and others are indicated.

CEREBRAL PALSY

A relatively common group of neurological problems which are encountered during evaluations of children with developmental delays are the cerebral palsies. Most often cerebral palsy is secondary to a static intracranial neurological impairment which commonly is associated with prematurity, intracranial hemorrhage, hypoxia, and kernicterus. Cerebral palsy is defined as a non-progressive disorder (static encephalopathy) of movement and posture due to brain insult or injury, occurring in the period of early brain growth and development (including the prenatal period through early childhood to three to five years of age). Different clinical signs representative of the underlying brain damage may appear throughout motor development.

The most common symptom associated with cerebral palsy is a delay in motor development such as rolling over, sitting, standing, crawling, or walking. Other early symptoms of cerebral palsy include: excessive irritability (constant crying and sleeping difficulties); feeding problems (difficulties in sucking, swallowing, chewing, spitting up); jitteriness; excessive startle reactions to noises and changes in posture; stiffness of the body which make it difficult to feed and bathe the infant; early standing due to hypertonia; and a definite hand preference during the first 18 months of life.

On physical examination, the physician may find signs of an intracranial lesion such as those described previously; however, more commonly nothing specific will be found. On the neurological examination of infants with cerebral palsy, there will probably be delays in motor development and delays on the Milani Comparetti examination. For instance, primary motor patterns may persist when they should be disappearing, and/or there may be a delay in the onset of or asymmetry in some of the motor patterns (such as head control and/or the parachute reactions).

The more traditional neurologic signs of cerebral palsy in children are generally seen at an older age—namely, between approximately a year-and-one-half and six years of age. On the neurological examination, the physician will find either hypotonia or hypertonia, as well as an increase in the reflexes, up-going toes, ankle clonus, and long tract signs. These findings may be limited to the limbs of the lower extremities or to one side of the body. Though there are names given to patterns of sites of involvement, these will not be discussed in this chapter since the physician is not being asked to make a specific diagnosis. Instead, the physician is expected to identify cases of cerebral palsy and to know what to do about them. (More detailed information about cerebral

palsy can be learned from a standard neurological text, or from one of the articles listed in the Bibliography which accompanies this chapter.)

It is important for the physician to realize that although some children with cerebral palsy also manifest intellectual impairment, many are intellectually normal. Therefore, it is extremely important that a child with early manifestations of cerebral palsy not be labeled mentally retarded when an accurate reflection of the child's intellectual development has not been obtained. Instead, the physician should follow the child and obtain psychological evaluations of the child's intellectual status at appropriate intervals.

It is generally agreed that infants and children manifesting cerebral palsy should be referred to physical or occupational therapists for two main reasons. The first is to teach or facilitate functional development of normal movement patterns, and the second is to prevent the development of contractures and deformities. Professionals working with children who have cerebral palsy are of the firm opinion that the earlier these children are identified and treated, the better the outcome. A common misconception is that treatment should not be started until a diagnosis is conclusively made. This does not take into account the fact that parents of cerebral palsied children also need assistance in dealing with the feeding, handling, sleeping, and temperament problems that so often accompany the condition. No doubt the reason why primary care physicians often fail to refer such children for treatment is due to the physicians' mistaken assumption that nothing can be done to assist these children and their families. Nothing can be further from the truth.

There have been many philosophies of the approach to these children, but in recent years therapy has been dominated internationally by the neurodevelopmental treatment approach of the Bobaths. In the normal developmental sequence, there is an evolutionary integration of the early primitive reflexes, and they are gradually brought under the influence of higher centers of control. In such a way, postural reactions gradually appear. These processes and their interrelationships are the basis of understanding the Bobath approach, and enable the application of these concepts to the treatment of infants and children with cerebral palsy or other movement disorders.

The neurodevelopmental rationale is that treatment techniques aimed at inhibition of patterns of abnormal reflex activity and the facilitation of normal motor patterns positively affect the motor development of these children. If these techniques are begun early and there are no interfering fixed contractures or preceding orthopedic procedures, treatment then becomes a combination of inhibition and facilitation by using special handling techniques.

MINOR MOTOR SEIZURES

An infrequent cause of delays (especially in intellectual development) is minor motor seizures. These do not include grand mal seizures which are very evident and common in developmentally disabled children. Rather, this chapter is intended to alert the physician to signs of minor motor seizures such as infantile spasms, akinetic seizures, petit mal seizures, and psychomotor seizures. It is beyond the scope of this chapter to teach the physician how to differentiate these types of seizures and how to treat them; rather, it is the aim here to teach the physician to recognize children manifesting such seizures.

The symptoms that should alert the physician to minor motor seizure disorders are poor attention span, decreased comprehension, staring spells, inappropriate pauses in speech, unusual facial movements, seemingly preprogrammed repetitive or perseverative movements, and sudden alterations in body posture or tone.

Signs on the examination which indicate a possible seizure disorder are signs of cerebral dysgenesis (including microcephaly), and skin lesions which might be indicative of a neurocutaneous disorder such as tuberous sclerosis; these are discussed further in Chapter 10. Unfortu-

nately, the neurological examination is always not helpful in diagnosing all children with a seizure disorder. If the physician suspects petit mal seizures, he or she may be able to elicit such a seizure by asking the patient to hyperventilate. If the history is suggestive of a seizure disorder, the physician may wish to order an electroencephalogram.

If a child is suspected of having any of the minor motor seizure disorders, it is recommended that referral be made to a neurologist, preferably a child neurologist, to evaluate the child more thoroughly and consider what treatment may be indicated.

PERIPHERAL NEUROPATHY

Peripheral neuropathy may be due to a variety of conditions including toxic metabolic disease, Guillain-Barre syndrome, Werdnig-Hoffman infantile muscular atrophy, and heredito-familial diseases or degenerative disorders.

The symptoms and signs of peripheral neuropathy obviously will depend upon which nerves are involved. Thus, it may be that the physician will find isolated or mixed dysfunction involving motor, sensory, and/or autonomic pathways. Generally, the mental status is intact and the patient shows hyporeflexia in the involved area. Often there is a distal extremity weakness which frequently is bilateral, especially when the peripheral neuropathy is due to a toxic origin. Another finding is the weakness and atrophy of muscle. When the autonomic nervous system is involved, there may be decreased sweating and changes in the vasomotor tone.

It is recommended that if a child with peripheral neuropathy is identified, that referral should be made to a neurologist.

MUSCLE DISEASE

The next condition that will be discussed encompasses the various muscle diseases that may be encountered. These as a whole are quite rare; however, they should be kept in mind as the physician evaluates a child who seems to be slow in motor development or who manifests signs of hypotonia.

The symptoms of muscle disease are delays or regressions in motor milestones, much as might be seen in the case of cerebral palsy. The young child may have trouble getting into the standing position and have to "walk" the hands up the body in order to right him- or herself. Generally, however, muscle diseases start after infancy with a gradual onset and often there is a positive family history of similar muscle disease, so that diagnosis should not be difficult. The signs include weakness, particularly in the proximal limb muscles. Sometimes the muscles which are involved may appear to be en-larged, but actually are quite weak. Sensation and intellectual function generally remain intact. Bowel and bladder function and deep tendon reflexes are usually relatively well preserved. The differential diagnosis of muscle disease would be muscular dystrophy, myasthenia gravis, dermatomyositis, periodic paralysis, and endocrine disorders such as hypothyroidism.

It is recommended that any time a child with probable muscle disease is encountered, referral should be made to the nearest muscle disease clinic. If such a clinic is not available, it is recommended that the child should be referred to a neurologist.

TABLE 8-1   Neurological Disorders

Problem	Symptoms (History)	Signs (Physical, Neuromotor, And Neurological Examinations)	Differential Diagnosis
Intracranial Lesion	Headaches, nausea, vomiting, lethargy, enlarging head, stiff neck	Microcephaly, megacephaly, papilledema, retinal hemorrhage, blurred vision, enlarged blind spot, optic atrophy, transillumination, cranial nerve signs	Subdural hematoma, abscess, tumor, hydrocephalus, CNS dysgenesis, cerebellar cyst
Cerebral Palsy	Delayed motor development (non-progressive), possible seizure disorders, excessive irritability, feeding problems, jitteriness, excessive startle, body stiffness, (precocious) hand preference	Primitive reflex (delayed appearance and disappearance), slow motor development, delays on Milani Comparetti, increased or decreased tone, Babinski present, ankle clonus	Intracranial mass, muscular dystrophy, peripheral neuropathy, degenerative disorder
Minor Motor Seizures	Poor attention and comprehension, staring spells, pauses in speech, facial movements, repetitive movements, lapses in body posture	Microcephaly, congenital malformations, skin lesions (tuberous sclerosis), development delayed, focal or lateralized signs	Types: infantile spasms, akinetic seizures, petit mal seizures, psychomotor seizures
Peripheral Neuropathy and Lower Motor Neuron Lesions	Sensory, motor, and/or autonomic dysfunction	Intellect intact, DTR decreased, weakness symmetrical or in area of nerve distribution, muscle atrophy, decreased sweat and vasomotor tone	Toxic and metabolic disorders, post-infectious disorders, arteritis, Werdnig-Hoffman, heredito-familial disorders, degenerative disorders
Muscle Disease	Delayed motor development, weakness, muscle cramps, stiffness, gradual onset, family history positive	Greater weakness proximal than distal, sensation intact, bowel and bladder okay, DTR okay, sometimes pseudohypertrophy	Muscular dystrophy, myasthenia gravis, dermatomyositis, periodic paralysis, endocrine disturbance
Degenerative Disorders	Arrest in acquisition of intellectual and motor milestones, regression in skills	Intellect deterioration, possible seizures, spasticity, Babinski positive, central blindness, deafness, systemic manifestations	Intracranial mass, hydrocephalus, toxic disorders, minor motor seizures, meningitis, encephalitis

DEGENERATIVE DISORDERS

Fortunately, the degenerative disorders are extremely rare; unfortunately, they are generally not treatable. Nevertheless, it is important for the physician to identify such degenerative disorders as specifically as possible for family counseling purposes.

The hallmark symptom of degenerative disorders is an arrest in the development of a child, or regression in previously-acquired skills. The specific symptoms will naturally depend upon the type of degenerative disorder and its pathological nature. Signs—just as the symptoms—depend upon the type of degenerative disorder, the etiology, and the site of the lesion.

It is recommended that anytime a child is suspected of having a degenerative disorder, he or she should be promptly referred to a neurologist.

SUMMARY

This chapter has reviewed some of the more common neurological disorders which may be encountered during evaluation of children who are suspect on developmental screening. Although this list is far from complete, these include microcephaly, intracranial lesions, cerebral palsy, inapparent seizures or minor motor seizures, peripheral neuropathy, muscle disease, and degenerative disorders.

Table 8-1 summarizes these disorders, their signs, symptoms, and recommendations for treatment.

This chapter also has discussed several important points regarding procedures to use during the evaluation of suspect children. First, the physician should gather appropriate data through the history, the medical examination, the neuromotor developmental examination, and the neurological examination. Second, the signs and symptoms of neurological disorders should be identified, for these may explain the cause of a child's slowness in development. Finally, this chapter has discussed indications for referral for a more extensive evaluation by a neurologist. It has not discussed indications for specific sophisticated neurological investigations (such as the CAT scan), because in general, if a child has problems severe enough to warrant further evaluation, that child should be referred.

In summary, the vast majority of children who manifest delays in development will not have obvious signs of neurological disorders. However, these signs may be identified if they are carefully sought. It is expected that the primary care physician will be able to identify children who have serious neurological disorders, will be able to make appropriate referrals for further evaluation and/or treatment, and will participate in the ongoing process of explanation and counseling of the child's parents.

APPENDIX A

The Milani Comparetti Motor Development Screening Test*

OBJECTIVES

This manual and the videotape recording entitled "The Milani-Comparetti Motor Development Screening Test" have been prepared to provide instruction in Milani-Comparetti test procedures and scoring methods. After studying this material, the reader should be able to:

1. Name the key ages for administration of the test.
2. Perform the test procedures, with practice.
3. Identify normal and deviant responses to test procedures.
4. Mark appropriate scores on the forms provided.

INTRODUCTION

The physically handicapped child requires special instruction so that he can learn to take full advantage of the abilities he has. The sooner handicaps are detected, the sooner the child can begin to receive the special training which can help him lead a more productive life.

The Milani-Comparetti Motor Development Test is a series of simple procedures designed to evaluate a child's motor development from birth to about two years of age. Using this test, a physician, therapist, nurse, or physician's assistant can determine in minutes whether one child's motor development corresponds to that of a normal child. When administered several times over a period of months, the test indicates trends in a child's motor development. This information can be used to identify a need for more detailed developmental evaluation.

The attractiveness of the Milani-Comparetti test lies in its simplicity. This test can be conducted effectively on an examining table or floor area with no special equipment. It can be easily and unobtrusively incorporated into the child's routine physical examinations. For children under 12 months of age, repeated examinations are especially valuable in establishing that a problem exists, since developmental problems detected early can be treated early.

The test may be most helpful if conducted at specific intervals. Key ages appropriate for testing are:

1½ to 2 months	15 months
3½ to 4 months	18 months
5½ to 6 months	21 months
9 to 10 months	24 months
12 months	

---

*Excerpted with the permission of Meyer Children's Rehabilitation Institute, University of Nebraska Medical Center, Omaha, Nebraska, copyright 1977, Project Director: Jack Trembath, M.B., B.S., M.R.C. Psych., F.A.A.P.

More frequent testing may be indicated for the child who shows consistent delays, asymmetry, or other abnormal motor development.

Generally, professionals or parents assess a child's level of physical motor, intellectual, social and emotional development by comparing the child's behavior and performance with generally recognized "norms." Yet, it is impossible to say that any behavior is normal or abnormal in all circumstances. Because motor development occurs gradually, there can be no absolute determinations that a given response is normal or abnormal for a particular age. Nevertheless, the concept of "normal" is valuable in providing grounds upon which to base judgments and subsequent actions. There may well be no cause for alarm if a child deviates slightly from what is indicated as normal, but a persistent deviation can point up a need for additional attention in a particular area.

Behavior or responses which deviate significantly from the normal are possible, and they can be serious. If such deviations do appear, or if deviations persist over an extended time, the examiner should request more extensive tests to confirm or deny any apparent abnormality.

MILANI-COMPARETTI TEST PROCEDURES

Originally, Milani-Comparetti and Gidoni presented their testing procedure and scoring chart with the statement that further modification might be beneficial after use and review by other professionals. The Meyer Children's Rehabilitation Institute staff has developed the modification presented here to permit smoother, more rapid administration of the test. All of the original test procedures and scoring mechanisms are retained; they are simply placed in a different order for more efficient testing.

To assess the child's reflexes and degree of motor control, follow the procedures described in this section of the manual. Drawings are included to show the positions of the child for specific tests and the reactions of a normal child to given stimuli. The following section contains instructions for use of the scoring chart.

When testing, note the state of the child just before and during the exam. Is he alert, cooperative, or crying? Did he have to be awakened, or was his bottle taken away? Also note environmental influences such as the temperature of the room. Such factors may influence a child's responses. An irritable child may resist some of the test procedures. In such cases, you must rely on information provided by the person who brings the child for examination. You might indicate on the scoring sheet that a child was resistant and untestable on certain items. Future tests when the child is more cooperative may confirm or deny deviant findings.

Body Lying Supine

Lay the child on his back and observe the movement of his head. Normally, a child at 5 months of age lifts his head forward as he anticipates being pulled up to sitting (Figure 1).

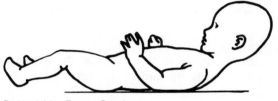

Figure 1. At 5 months, the baby voluntarily lifts his head from supine.

Body Pulled Up From Supine

While the child is in the supine position, grasp his forearms and gently pull him to a sitting position. As you pull, watch the child's head, neck and shoulders. Normal reactions, shown in Figure 2, are:

Younger than 4 months — head remains back or "lags" to varying degrees.
4 to 5 months — head is kept aligned with body.
5 months or older — the head leads the body, and the shoulders and arms flex in an effort to collaborate with the examiner.

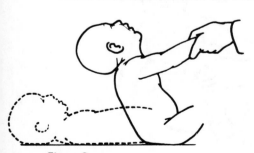
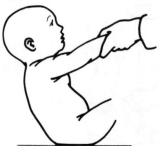
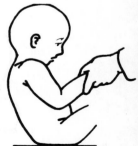

Figure 2.
Younger than 4 months, the head lags behind the body.

4 to 5 months, child keeps head in line with the body.

5 months or older, head leads the body.

Sitting Posture

Place the child in the sitting position and look at the curvature of his back. The line drawings on the scoring chart give guidelines to expected development at different ages. Normal responses are:

Younger than 4 months — completely rounded back.

4 months — extension or straightening of back to the level of the third lumbar segment (indicated by L3 on the chart).

6 months — extension or straightening upper and lower back, and propping forward with hands.

7 months — sitting independently without propping, though posture may be unsteady.

8 months — sitting erect with no difficulty.

Sideways Parachute

Parachute reactions are protective responses to sudden disruption of balance.
A parachute response is an automatic extension of the limbs.

THE BABY MUST HAVE GOOD HEAD CONTROL BEFORE ANY OF THE PARACHUTE RESPONSES ARE TESTED.

To check the sideways parachute response, begin with the child in the sitting position, holding him firmly at the waist. Quickly but firmly tip him to the side to see whether he extends his arm to catch himself as his balance is disrupted.

After the age of 6 months, a normal child tries to protect himself from falling by extending his arm and open hand, as shown in Figure 3. This reaction is usually not seen before the age of 6 months.

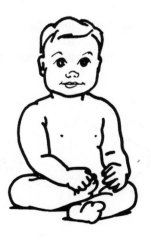
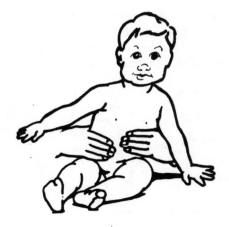

Figure 3.

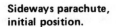

Sideways parachute,
initial position.

Normal reaction

Backwards Parachute

Again holding the child in a sitting position, tip him gently backwards. Usually a child 9 months or older reacts to the sudden imbalance by either extending both hands behind him or rotating to one side to catch himself with his hand. (Figure 4).

Do not test this reaction in a child who does not have good head control to avoid rapid flexion and extension of the neck.

Figure 4.

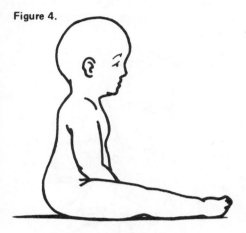

Figure 4A. Initial testing position, backwards parachute

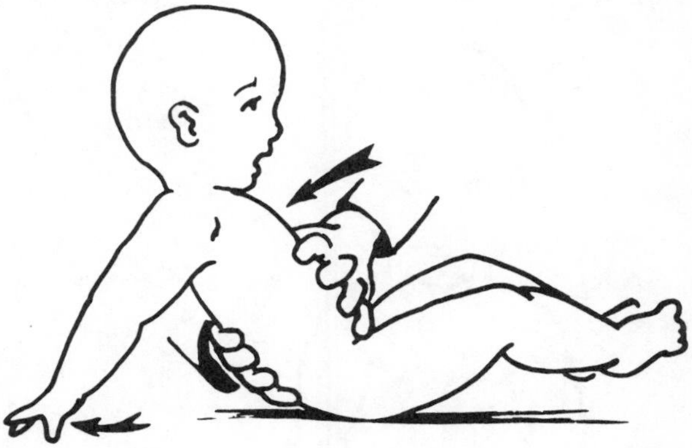

Figure 4B. Normal reaction, extending both arms backward.

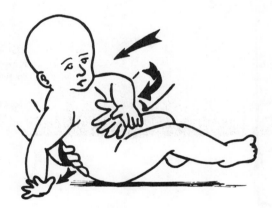

Figure 4C. Normal reaction, turning to one side

Body Held Vertical

This is one of several procedures designed to demonstrate the ability of the child to control his head. Place your hands at mid-trunk level well below the axilla to prevent shoulder elevation. Lift the child to a vertical position with his legs suspended in the air. Note the position of the child's head. A 1-month-old child is usually unable to control his head, but gradually, by the age of 4 months, he develops full head control, maintaining the head in midline.

Head in Space

Continuing to hold the child in vertical suspension, tilt him slowly first to the left, then to the right. Continue tilting him slowly forward, then backward Be careful not to let the head fall back suddenly. For an infant with poor head control or a premature newborn, be careful to prevent hyperextension of the neck when tilting the child backward.

When tilted, the child should try to adjust his head so that it remains upright regardless of body position, with the eyes and mouth horizontal and the nose vertical. Observations indicate that this reaction normally begins to appear at about 1½ months of age and is complete by 4 months. Figure 5 shows head in space reactions.

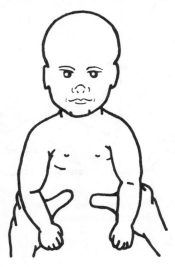

Figure 5A
Initial testing position,
head in space

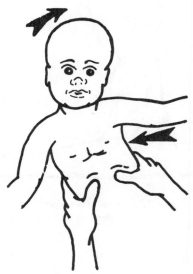

Figure 5B
Normal reaction
to sideways tilting.

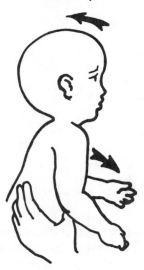

Figure 5C.
Normal reaction
to forward tilting.

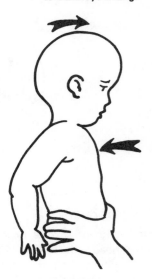

Figure 5D.
Normal reaction
to backward tilting.

Downward Parachute

The test for the downward parachute response should be attempted only after the child has demonstrated head control.

First lift the child vertically some distance from the examination table. Once his legs are somewhat flexed, lower him rapidly 2 to 3 feet so that he gets the feeling of falling. If no response is elicited by lowering to the table top, lower the child to the floor. The normal child at about 4 months of age reacts by straightening and spreading his legs and turning his feet outward (Figure 6).

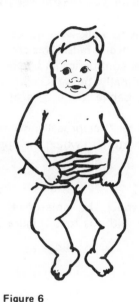

Figure 6

Initial testing position, downward parachute.

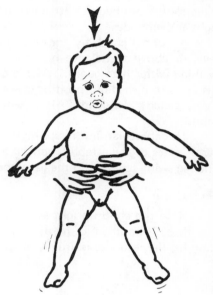

Normal response

Standing

To test the child's ability to stand, hold him upright above the examining table. Then lower him slowly so that his feet touch the table. Notice whether the child can support his weight well. Normal development of this ability is:

5 months — able to support own weight; legs are semi-flexed.
8 months — able to stand with support, with trunk slightly forward and hips flexed.
10 months — able to stand erect with support.
12 months — able to stand independently.

The shaded area of the chart represents primitive supporting reactions present at birth but absent by about 2½ months of age. Test for these primitive supporting reactions by holding the child upright and letting his feet touch the top of the table so that he supports at least part of his weight. Usually a child younger than 2½ months immediately stiffens his legs in extension. This is called "positive supporting." If the child is between 2½ and 5 months of age, his legs may collapse as you lower him toward the table. This inability to support weight is called "astasia," as noted on the scoring chart.

Locomotion

If the child can support his own weight stiffly, try to elicit a stepping reaction by shifting his weight slightly from side to side and tilting him forward. Automatic stepping usually disappears when the child is 1½ to 2 months old.

Next, let the child lie on his back, preferably on the floor, and observe his movements. At the age of 4 to 6 months, a child can usually roll over. If rolling is not observed in the exam, ask the mother whether the child rolls from stomach to back (the usual first direction), from back to stomach, or from back to side. Determine whether he rolls to both right and left sides.

A normal child, by approximately 12 months, begins to walk with hands at shoulder level or above to balance himself and to protect himself from falls. This stance is called walking with "high guard." As the child matures, he gains confidence and gradually lowers his arms to a medium position, called "medium guard." Finally, he walks with hands at his sides, called "no guard." This sequence usually occurs between the ages of 12 and 21 months.

The abbreviation "recip. mvts." on the chart stands for "reciprocal movements." The term refers to the establishment of a more advanced gait pattern in which the opposite arm and leg swing together in the gait sequence.

Foot Grasp

Hold the child upright at the trunk so that his feet touch the tabletop. If the child is less than 9 months old, he usually grasps at the tabletop with his toes (Figure 7). After 9 months, the response is usually absent.

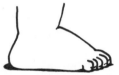

Figure 7   **Between birth and 9 months, the toes grasp when the foot contacts a surface.**

Body in Sagittal Plane (Landau Response)

Suspend the child in a prone position by supporting him under the upper abdomen with the palm of your hand, as shown in Figure 8. Note the position of the child's head, trunk and legs. Normally, a child from the age of 2 to 3 months onward tries to straighten his body. This extension develops cephalocaudally, and is usually complete at 4 to 6 months. By 6 to 7 months or older, the child can voluntarily inhibit the response.

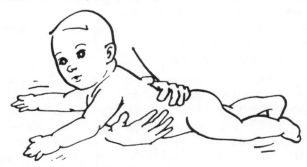

Figure 8   **Child suspended in the prone position.**

Forward Parachute

Like the other parachute reactions, this should not be tested until the child has demonstrated head control!

Hold the child firmly at mid-trunk level, with his back to you. Suspend him vertically above the table, then tilt him forward suddenly. A normal child reacts by straightening his arms in front of him and extending his fingers (Figure 9). You may observe this reaction in children as young as 7 months. Asymmetry in the upper extremities can be detected in this maneuver.

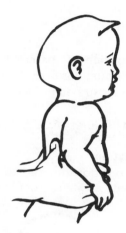
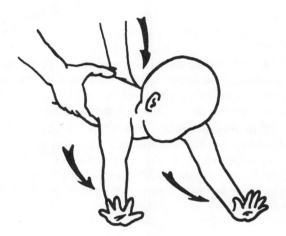

Figure 9A.   Initial testing
position,
forward parachute.

Figure 9B.
Normal reaction.

Body Lying Prone

Lay the child on his stomach and again watch for head movement. Figure 10 shows the degree of head control that a child should be able to demonstrate at 2, 4 and 6 months of age.

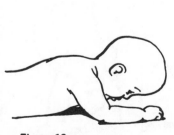
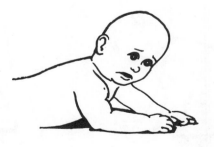
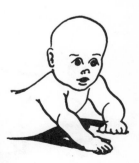

Figure 10

2 months — head in line
with body.

4 months — head elevated
about 45 degrees

6 months — head elevated
about 90 degrees

Hand Grasp

With the child lying prone, be sure that his hands are touching the examination table. Until the age of about 3½ months, the child's hand assumes the fisted position while it is in contact with the tabletop (Figure 11).

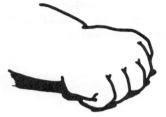

Figure 11

**Hand grasp response,
normal until age 3½ months.**

All Fours

"All fours" as listed on the chart, refers not to the position of the child for the examination, but rather to the child's ability to assume the all-fours position. To evaluate this category of postural control, lay the child on his stomach. As illustrated in Figure 12, the pattern of motor development in this area is normally:

3½ months — Child is able to support part of his weight on his forearms.

5 months — Child is able to support himself on his hands.

7 to 9 months — Child can assume the hands and knees position.

10 to 12 months — Child can assume a hands-and-feet position referred to on the scoring chart as "plantigrade." This later develops into the ability to stand from the center of the floor.

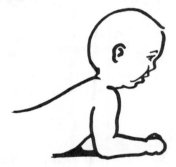

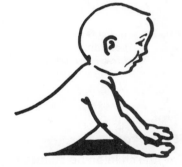

**Figure 12   3½ months — child
props on forearms.**

**5 months — child supports
self on hands.**

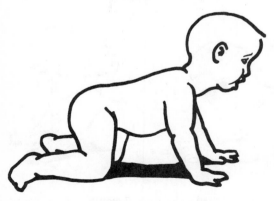

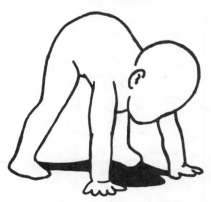

**7 to 9 months — child
on hands and knees.**

**10 to 12 months — child in
plantigrade position on
hands and feet.**

Symmetric Tonic Neck Reflex

If you are testing a child older than 6 months, place him in the all fours crawling position. Then, with your hand on his forehead, gently lift his head while supporting him under the trunk. The symmetric tonic neck reflex is seen when the child flexes hips and knees under him as if to sit on his feet, while extending his neck and arms (Figure 13). This reflex disappears when the child can lift his buttocks from his heels without flexing his neck or arms, or when he is able to crawl reciprocally on hands and knees.

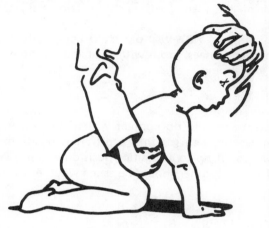

Figure 13

Body Derotative

"Derotation," as the term implies, means untwisting. Place the child in the supine position and flex one hip and knee across his body in a motion similar to cranking. A child younger than 4 months "log rolls," with the body rolling as a unit. After 4 months, the child actively untwists segmentally to the prone position. (Figure 14)

The body derotative response should be tested both to the right and left.

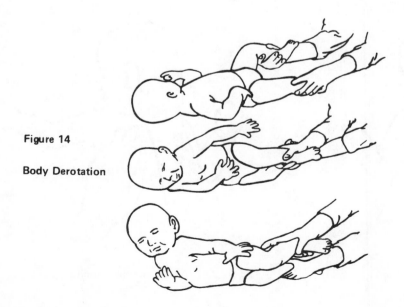

Figure 14

Body Derotation

Standing Up From Supine

With the mother standing nearby to reassure the child and to act as a motivator, place the child supine on a covered floor. From this position, a normal 9- to 11-month old child rolls over onto his stomach and pulls himself to standing, using either his mother or objects in the room for support.

At 12 to 15 months, the child should be able to stand without the aid of objects. He does this by first assuming a position on hands and feet with buttocks resting on his heels. Then he lifts his hips, assuming the plantigrade position, and straightens into a standing position, all without support.

When standing up from supine, a 3½-year-old child commonly partially rotates the trunk on the pelvis, flexes hips and knees, props with the hand on the side toward which he has rotated, and then comes to standing.

Body Rotative

The body rotative reactions require no contact with the child. A child 9 months or older performs a series of movements to get into a different position. At 9 months, the child, upon awakening, pulls himself up to a standing position in the crib. Since this cannot be observed in the examination, the mother should be asked whether the child pulls to stand in the crib.

Asymmetric Tonic Neck Reflex (ATNR)

First, place the child on his back. Keeping his neck in line with his body and stablizing his trunk with one hand, gently turn his head to one side. Holding this position for about 10 seconds, watch the child's arms. When the head is turned to the left, for example, a normal infant responds by flexing his right elbow and straightening the left arm as shown in Figure 15. The relative increase in flexion of the arm on the skull side shows the presence of the response.

The ATNR is usually present in infants 1 to 4 months old.

Figure 15

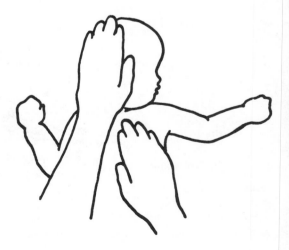

ATNR, initial position   ATNR, normal response

Moro Reflex

The procedure described here is modified from the original description to avoid any unnecessary sudden extension of the baby's neck.

Cradle the child in a semi-reclined position of about 45 degrees. Be sure to support his head with your hand. Keeping your hand and forearm under his head and trunk, quickly drop his entire body downward and back. The sudden loss of support should produce a good Moro response without letting the baby's head fall back unsupported.

The baby responds by extending his arms from the body and quickly opening his hands and fingers (Figure 16). This maneuver is excellent for early detection of asymmetry in the upper extremities. The response should disappear at approximately 4 months of age.

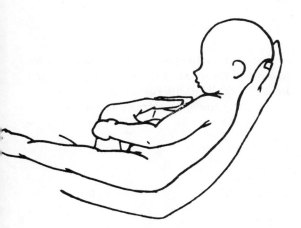
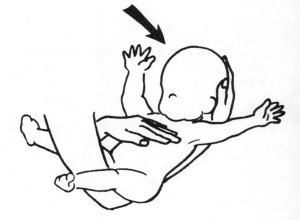

Figure 16A.
Initial position
for testing Moro
reflex.

Figure 16B.
Moro reflex.
Extended arms, open hands
and fingers.

Tilting Reactions

The final group of reactions, the tilting reactions, are not routinely tested in office examinations because they require the use of a tilt board or a table that can be tilted. Certainly, the tilting reactions should be evaluated in any examination which appears questionable or in which there is a suspicion of abnormal motor development. In these reactions, the examiner should note curving of the spine only. Reactions of the limbs are not significant in the tilting procedures on young children, since limb reactions are difficult to distinguish from those of similar parachute reactions.

In the drawings that follow, stick figures are used to illustrate the curvature of the trunk in these reactions.

Prone Tilting Reaction

Lay the child on his stomach, and carefully raise one side of the table. The normal child tries to compensate by curving his spine with the concavity toward the raised side of the table (Figure 17). The arms and legs should abduct away from the body. Conduct this test so that the child curves his spine first to one side and then to the other.

The reaction usually appears in children 5 months and older.

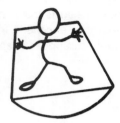

Figure 17
Prone Tilting Reaction

Supine Tilting Reaction

Turn the child over onto his back. Lift the edge of the table parallel to the child's side. He should again attempt to compensate by curving his spine up toward the raised side of the table, with extremities extending outward (Figure 18). Test both the right and left sides.

The ability to curve the spine in the supine position usually appears at about 7 months of age.

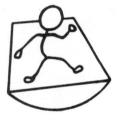

Figure 18
Supine Tilting Reaction

Sitting Tilting Reaction

Place the child in a sitting position on the table with his back to you. Lift the edge of the table first on one side, then the other. Again, the normal child tries to compensate by curving his spine sideways with the concavity toward the raised side and extending extremities away from the body (Figure 19).

The sitting tilting reaction develops later than either the prone or the supine reaction. It is unlikely that a child younger than 7 months will demonstrate this reaction. The reaction usually begins to appear around 7 months and is not fully developed until 8 months.

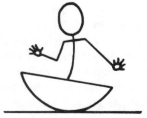

Figure 19
Sitting Tilting Reaction

All Fours Tilting Reaction

Place the child on all fours facing you and tilt the table slowly from side to side. A normal child reacts by curving his spine with the concavity toward the raised side of the table (Figure 20). Again, be sure to test in both directions. Normally, a child between the ages of 8 and 12 months begins to show signs of reacting to this test.

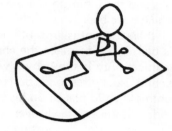

Figure 20
All Fours Tilting Reaction

Standing Tilting Reaction

As the child stands unsupported on the table with his back to you, carefully lift one side of the table. Watch the child closely to see whether he curves his spine, again with the concavity toward the raised side, to compensate for the tilted surface. (Figure 21).

The standing reaction develops even more gradually than the sitting and all fours tilting reactions. The standing reaction begins to appear at 12 months and is usually fully developed by the age of 21 months.

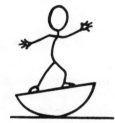

Figure 21
Standing Tilting Reaction

FURTHER NOTES ON TEST PROCEDURES

Testing the Older Child

In their original articles, Milani-Comparetti and Gidoni stated that the testing of a child may commence at the level of motor development that the child has attained. This is based on the assumption that the child reaches higher stages of development through the emergence of some responses and the inhibition of others. Therefore, it is unnecessary to go back and retest responses which have been previously acquired or inhibited.

In testing a child older than 8 months who has acquired some of the basic locomotor skills, we ask the mother's permission to place the child on a rug on the examining room floor. (Of course, this is practical only if the baby is well and the exam room is not a clinic area for sick children.) The child usually responds better on the floor than on a table.

For example, a 10-month-old child placed on his back on the floor usually rolls over to his stomach, gets up on hands and knees, crawls over to his mother, and pulls up to stand at her knee. If the child is put on the floor in a sitting position, his sitting posture as well as change of positions can be seen.

The motor skills observed in such a situation are many of those higher skill levels represented in the Milani-Comparetti test. If the examiner has any doubts about the way the child moves, then testing particular areas is warranted. For instance, if a child shows asymmetrical use of his limbs when getting up at his mother's knee, it would be appropriate to test the sideways, forward, downward and backward parachute responses. If there is any question regarding the development or disappearance of an early response, its test can easily be incorporated into the examination. Generally, this is not necessary if the child has no apparent difficulty in his ability to perform the higher levels of postural control and movement.

When to Omit Tests

A baby should not be put through test procedures above his chronological age when it is obvious that his motor development and age level are not near the age level of the expected response. Generally, we have omitted test items that are in a 1- to 1½-month range above the baby's chronological age. Also, if the baby appears to be generally behind his age level, as is often true of premature infants, we have tried to keep the testing routines within the developmental level of the child.

For example, the sideways parachute reactions are not tested in a 4½-month-old child, since these responses do not usually appear until 6 months. A premature child of 6 months who had been born 2 months early also would not be tested for parachute reactions in most situations.

Each infant is different, so the examiner must make some decisions as to when to test the individual baby for particular test items. The stick figures, words, and shaded areas on the chart provide basic guidelines for the expected age levels at which various responses may be expected.

Obviously, it is not necessary to test a child for responses far below his age level if he appears to be progressing well in motor skills and responses.

SCORING THE MILANI-COMPARETTI MOTOR DEVELOPMENT TEST

THE CHART

The scoring chart is a graphic profile of a child's motor development. The sample chart to be used with this manual is found in Appendix B.

The first 12 months on the chart are divided by vertical lines into one-half month increments. The appropriate age in months appears directly above the vertical line. From 12 to 24 months, the chart is condensed into a shorter scale; each vertical line represents 1 month.

The shaded areas on the chart represent the time span when a reflex or reaction is expected to be present. The tapered shaded areas (appearing in the tilting reactions) indicate that these responses emerge gradually within the tapered period.

Unshaded tapered arrows (in the body held vertical and body lying prone tests) indicate that the motor reaction being tested — head control — is acquired gradually.

The stages of development depicted by the stick figures on the chart are explained in the procedures section of this manual. Their positions on the chart serve as guidelines to show the age levels at which postural changes occur in motor development.

In the words printed on the chart, the first letter is aligned vertically with the age at which that motor skill or response usually appears.

The chart used to test a child initially may also be used to score later tests so that relative gains or delays with age can be readily assessed. The date when each test is given is written above the number in months which corresponds to the child's chronological age. However, in testing high-risk babies, a new chart should be used for each test, so that the examiner cannot be influenced by the results of previous tests. Results of all tests may then be combined and transferred to a single form.

Often it is helpful to prepare a narrative summary of special observations made at each testing session. The narratives may be attached to the back of the profile chart for the child, and thus provide a continuing summary of that child's motor development. Examples of some of the summaries prepared at the Meyer Children's Rehabilitation Institute are given in Appendix C.

General Scoring

The child's age in months is used to score each item tested. The scoring number thus remains the same throughout the test; a 5-month-old child will be scored entirely with 5's. The child's actual age is placed in the column corresponding to his performance on each test item. Thus, if a 5-month-old child performs at the 3-month level in one area, a 5 is written on the vertical line headed by the number 3.

In determining a child's age, no allowance is made for prematurity. The number of months since birth is accepted as the child's age for recording. However, length of gestation is considered when interpreting the significance of delays. Experience has shown that premature infants by the age of 10 to 15 months make gains to the point at which their level of development is equivalent to that of a term baby.

When scoring, it is best to avoid ambiguous terms such as "partial" and "incomplete." Most responses should be judged either as absent or present. The only exceptions are the test items indicated on the scoring sheet with tapered arrows, which show emerging reactions.

SCORING NORMAL RESPONSES

.If a child's response to a test item is the normal expected for his age, write the age on the vertical line headed by the same number, as shown below.

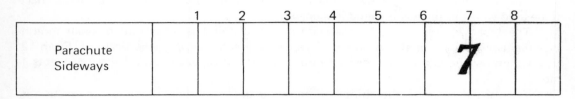

Several of the test items may be difficult to observe directly, especially if the child is uncooperative. In such a situation, the mother can often provide the necessary information. You might ask her such questions as, "Does your baby roll over yet? From his back to his tummy? From tummy to back?" and so on. The mother's answers may be entered on the chart with the notation "mother's report."

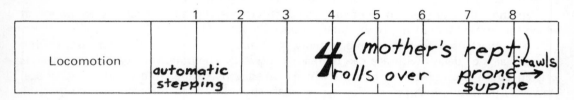

SCORING DEVIANT RESPONSES

When performing the test, you should be alert to deviations from the normal. Such deviations may include asymmetry, delay, advance, abnormalities within the response, or a combination of these.

In scoring deviations, place the child's actual age in months on the vertical line headed by the number of months at which the observed response normally occurs. Mark the number that you write with an asterisk. Examples of specific scoring methods are given below. The principles shown in these examples may be applied throughout the scoring.

I.   *Asymmetry*

Both sides of the body should respond equally to each test item. Symmetry should become particularly evident after the fourth month as the influence of the asymmetric tonic neck reflex disappears. However, symmetry can be seen earlier in testing the Moro response. As examples of normal symmetrical responses, the hands open equally in the Moro response, parachute responses prevent falling on both sides, and weight is distributed evenly over both legs in standing.

Examples of asymmetrical reactions, which may be indications of possible hemiplegia, may include a hand grasp or foot grasp on one side that persists beyond the normal time for disappearance, asymmetric posturing of the arms in the Moro response, an absent parachute response on one side, or unequal weight-bearing on one side of the body. A cluster of asymmetries may be more evidence of a problem in this area than is a single asymmetrical response in isolation.

A. Sideways Parachute

In the parachute responses, the child's reactions should be equal on both sides. If the response is present on one side but absent on the other, it should be scored as an asymmetrical response, marked with an asterisk and notation.

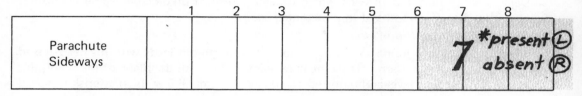

B. Head in Space

In the scoring shown in the chart below, the 4-month-old child righted his head when his body was tilted to his left. However, the response was incomplete when the body was tilted to his right. A 4 is placed on the line vertically aligned with 4 months, and the score is marked with an asterisk with notation made of the asymmetry.

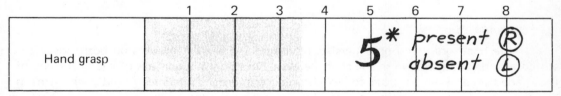

C. Hand Grasp

A 5-month-old infant normally does not exhibit a hand grasp response. For the child scored in the chart below, one hand demonstrated the appropriate absence of the hand grasp, but the response was present in the other hand. This is an asymmetrical reaction. Because the response on one side was appropriate for the child's age level, his age — 5 months — was placed in the column headed by 5. However, the 5 is marked with an asterisk, and notation is made that the response is present on one side and absent on the other.

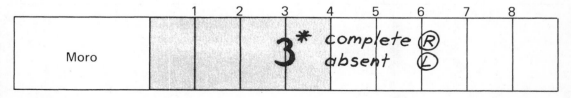

D. Moro

The Moro reflex is present until about 4 months of age. Extension and abduction of the arms with fully open hands should occur bilaterally. If not, the response is asymmetrical, and the scoring is again marked with an asterisk and a short explanation is made on the back of the chart.

			1	2	3	4	5	6	7	8
Moro					**3*** complete Ⓡ absent Ⓛ					

II.   *Delayed Responses*

Many reflexes which are normally present in the first few months of life disappear and become integrated or modified into more complex motor patterns. If a reflex persists 1 month beyond its normal time for disappearance, it signifies a delay in development.

Delay is also indicated if skills which usually appear at predictable age levels do not develop within 1 to 1½ months of that predicted age.

A. Body Pulled Up From Supine

When pulled from supine to sitting, a normal 5-month-old leads with his head flexed forward and pulls with his arms. If the head remains in line with the plane of the body, this is scored at the 4-month level and reported as a delay. A numeral 5 with an asterisk is placed on the sheet.

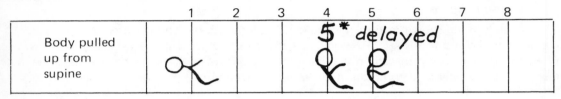

	1	2	3	4	5	6	7	8
Body pulled up from supine				5* delayed				

B. Sideways Parachute

The sideways parachute response should develop at 6 months. If it is absent on both sides for a 7-month-old, place a 7 in the column just outside the shaded area (in this case, at the 5½ month level). This means that the expected response is delayed and is not complete in either upper extremity. In such situations, score the item as close to the child's chronological age as possible.

	1	2	3	4	5	6	7	8
Parachute Sideways							7* delayed both sides	

C. Hand Grasp

If the hand grasp response persists beyond the age of 4 months on both sides, it is scored as a delay, as shown in the chart below. The child's actual age is placed at the end of the shaded area, again as close to his chronological age as possible. Avoid such terms as "partially open"; judge the response as either absent or present.

	1	2	3	4	5	6	7	8
Hand Grasp				6* delayed				

D. Asymmetrical Tonic Neck Reflex

The asymmetrical tonic neck posture normally disappears around the age of 4 months. If it is present in a 6-month-old, it represents a delay in modification of the reflex. Such a delay may prevent the child from rolling over. In scoring a delayed ATNR, the child's actual age is placed on the last vertical line which shows the response's existence.

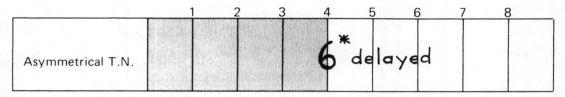

III. Advanced Responses

Occasionally, a child develops a skill before the predicted age level. A response is considered advanced if it appears 1 month or more before the expected age. Advanced responses are scored by writing the child's chronological age on the line headed by the number indicating when the response is expected. The score is marked with an asterisk to indicate a deviation from normal.

A. Sitting

Normally, a child is able to sit upright, propping himself up with his hands, at the age of 6 months. A 5-month-old who sits supporting himself is advanced in this motor skill. This is scored with a 5 placed on the vertical line headed by 6, and reported as advanced.

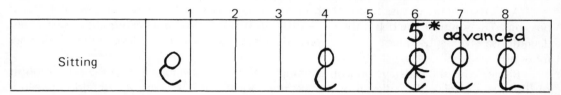

B. Locomotion

The chart below represents a 6½-month-old child who is already crawling on all fours. The child's age, 6.5, is placed at the beginning of the word "crawls," and his advanced development is noted with an asterisk.

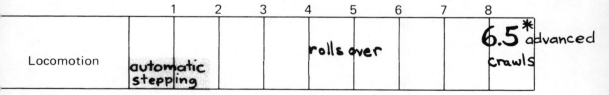

IV. *Combined Responses*

Retained and asymmetrical Moro response.

An example of combined deviations in responses to one test item is the child 6 months old who continues to show the Moro response, but consistently with the right hand fisted.

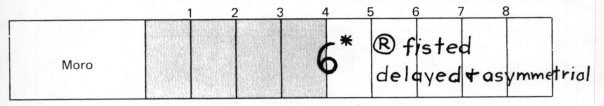

OTHER OBSERVATIONS

In testing babies with at-risk histories or babies of risk pregnancies, the examiner may see other behavior characteristics that are not part of the Milani-Comparetti screening test. The infant may show facial asymmetry in crying, a tremor in the hand, hypertonia or hypotonia.

Experience indicates that it is best *not* to note such observations on the scoring chart, so that the profile sheet shows only those items which have been specifically tested. However, it is useful to record such behaviors on another sheet which can be attached to the profile form. The attachment might also record limited observations about muscle tone, since it may show considerable variation among babies with differing histories.

An infant who is suspected of showing deviations should be tested several times if possible. The younger the baby, the more difficult it is to draw conclusions about significant deviations. Over subsequent test periods, delays or asymmetrical development becomes more obvious.

Babies who show delays and/or asymmetrical motor development in the early months of life may "catch up" or "even out" near the end of the first year. Any child between 9 and 12 months of age with significant delay and/or asymmetry should be watched closely with closely spaced retesting. Such a child should also be given a neurological evaluation and other developmental assessments. These will help to determine if the child's developmental status warrants early intervention with special training techniques. If so, the family also might be counseled and prepared to accept the idea of early management of the child's handicap, if one is identified.

SUMMARY

The Milani-Comparetti test can be used as a convenient and rapid screening test for motor development of children in the first two years of life. The test examines various stages of motor development in relation to the emergence and disappearance of primitive reflexes and also the sequential development of higher patterns of movement and postural control. We have found the Milani-Comparetti screening test convenient for the following reasons.

1. It can be easily incorporated into the routine office or clinical exam by physicians, therapists, nurses, or physicians' assistants.

2. It does not require specific equipment and thus can be easily administered in almost any type of setting.

3. It takes only a short time to administer (4 to 8 minutes), depending on the age of the child and the experience of the examiner.

4. It depends on predictable responses which are observed by the examiner as he handles the child to elicit these responses. It does not rely as much on the mother's history which may not be interpreted correctly.

5. It is scored graphically on a profile sheet for future comparison with subsequent retests.

The Milani-Comparetti test should be repeated several times during the child's first two years. Key ages recommended for examination are: 1½ – 2 months, 3½ – 4 months, 5½ – 6 months, 9 – 10 months, 12 months, 15 months, 18 months, 21 months, and 24 months. A baby who, in repeated testing, arouses suspicions because of consistent delays, asymmetry, abnormal development, or combinations of these deviations may warrant more frequent examination than the suggested intervals.

Since his physical and emotional state during the examination may influence a child's motor responses, the profile sheet should note the child's general state.

When a child has consistently shown deviant motor behavior on repeated examinations, or shown obviously abnormal responses, a thorough motor assessment and neurological examination should be considered.

CHART NO. 1 – ORIGINAL

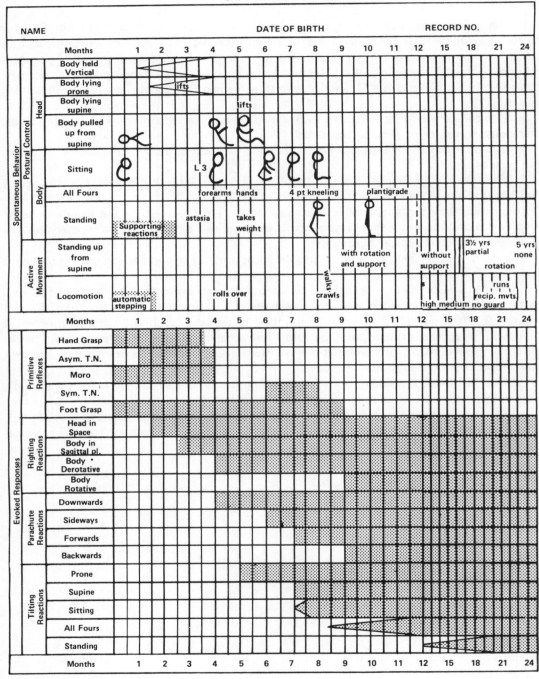

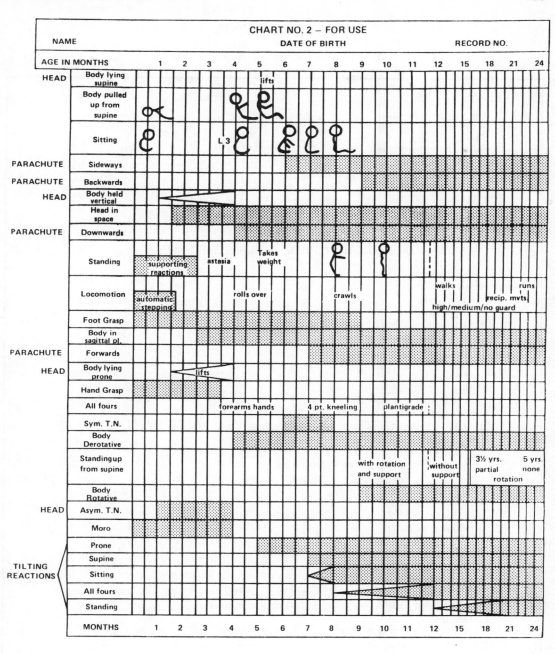

CHART NO. 2 – FOR USE

| NAME | | DATE OF BIRTH | RECORD NO. |

APPENDIX B

Neurological Examination Checklist

Name _____ Date _____

Mental Status
    Alert
    Explores environment
    Language comprehension
    Speech, reading, spelling, naming
    Intellect
    Visuomotor skills
    Stereognosis
    Graphesthesia
    Affect (sad, happy, appropriate, inappropriate)
    Performance characteristics (initiate, sustain, inhibit, shift)

Cranial Nerves
    Smell—I
    Visual fields—II
    Fundoscopic—II
    Pupillary size, shape, reactivity, color—III
    Extraocular movements—III, IV, VI
    Ptosis—III
    Jaw strength—V
    Corneal reflex—V
    Suck—V, XII
    Facial movements—VII
    Close eyes—VII
    Wrinkle forehead, smile, show teeth, purse lips—VII
    Gag, swallow—IX, X
    Tongue movement—XII
    Neck turning, shoulder elevation—XI

Motor Examination
    Bulk, tone, strength
    Asymmetry
        Right vs left
        Proximal vs distal
        Upper extremity vs lower extremity
    Postural control (abnormal, asymmetrical)
    Developmental reflexes
        Primitive reflexes (see Milani Comparetti)
        Acquired motor control (see Milani Comparetti)
    Handedness
    Developmental milestones (roll, sit, crawl, stand, walk, run, hop, bicycle)
    Fine motor coordination

Sensory
    Pin
    Touch
    Temperature
    Vibration
    Proprioception

Autonomic
    Vasomotor tone
    Sweating

Cerebellar
Finger-nose
Heel-shin
Rapid alternating movements
Hand pat
Foot tap
Retrieve objects
Trace lines
Touch between points

Gait and Balance
Normal
Tandem
Toes
Heels
Sides and feet
Stand on one foot
Hop

Deep Tendon Reflexes
Biceps
Triceps
Brachioradialis
Knee jerks
Ankle jerks

Abdominal Reflexes

Anal Sphincter Tone

Plantar Reflexes

Ankle Clonus

_____
Signature

BIBLIOGRAPHY

Barlow, C. F. Mental retardation and related disorders. *Contemporary Neurology Series,* 1978, *17* (whole volume).

Menkes, J. H. *Textbook of child neurology.* Philadelphia: Lea and Fehiger, 1974.

Milani-Comparetti, A. *Developmental prognosis.* Omaha: Meyer Children's Rehabilitation Institute, University of Nebraska Medical Center, 1979.

Milani-Comparetti, A., and Gidoni, E. A. Patterned analysis of motor development and its disorders. *Developmental Medicine and Child Neurology,* 1967, *9,* 625–630.

Neonatal Neurology. *Clinics in Perinatology,* 1977, *4* (whole volume).

Paine, R. S., and Oppe, T. E. Neurological examination of children. *Clinics in Developmental Medicine,* 1966, *20–21* (whole volume).

Pediatric Neurology. *Pediatric Clinics of North America,* 1976, *23* (whole volume).

Weiner, H., Bresnan, M., and Levitt, L. *Pediatric neurology for the house officer.* Baltimore: Williams and Wilkins, 1977.

Chapter 9

Goal   To develop skill in the recognition of inborn errors of metabolism that are
associated with retarded development, and to be aware of various types
of treatment for children with errors of metabolism.

Objectives   At the end of this chapter, the physician should be able to:
- explain the importance of early identification of inborn errors of
  metabolism;
- identify family history, signs, symptoms, and conventional laboratory
  data that are indicative of an inborn error of metabolism;
- state methods of confirming a metabolic diagnosis;
- state how to send laboratory specimens to confirm a metabolic diagnosis.

METABOLIC EVALUATION

By
DONOUGH O'BRIEN, M.D.
and EDWARD R. McCABE, M.D.

I. Introduction
   A. Inborn errors of metabolism are rare diseases individually, but collectively they are estimated at one per 1,000 children.
   B. Without accurate diagnosis of metabolic disorders, it is impossible to institute appropriate treatment.
II. Importance of Early Treatment
   A. Early treatment for metabolic disorders is necessary if mental retardation and other developmental problems are to be prevented or ameliorated.
   B. Appropriate treatment of maple syrup urine disease is essential within the first few weeks of life if life is to be sustained; early treatment of galactosemia can reverse cataracts and prevent mental retardation.
   C. Treatment of phenylketonuria begun within the first three weeks of life generally results in normal intellectual development; treatment delayed beyond the latter part of the first year usually results in irreparable mental retardation.
   D. The prognosis for intellectual development of infants with congenital hypothyroidism is directly related to the age at onset of treatment.
   E. Screening tests are not diagnostic; since they will inevitably fail to identify some children with metabolic disorders, it is essential to rule out these disorders through laboratory tests even when previous screening tests have been negative.
III. Implications for Genetic Counseling
   A. Information from antenatal diagnosis offers women the option of not continuing a pregnancy when it would inevitably result in a severely damaged child; in some cases, metabolic disorders can be diagnosed in the heterozygous state.
   B. Genetic counseling can prevent both the psychological grief and economic costs associated with having an affected child.
IV. Types of Metabolic Disorders
   A. Aminoacidopathies include phenylketonuria, cystinuria, and methylmalonic aciduria.
   B. Disorders of carbohydrate metabolism include galactosemia and glycogen storage diseases.
   C. Because many lysosomal storage diseases lead to severe clinical handicaps, carrier detection is important.
V. Identification of Metabolic Disorders
   A. The Metabolic Screening Checklist includes a family history which can be a diagnostic aid to the physician.
   B. Historic information to be noted includes: a history of fetal wastage; similar presentations and courses in siblings; knowledge of infant deaths; consanguinity; ethnic background; and other relatives with similar diseases.

VI. Symptoms Which Indicate a Possible Metabolic Disorder
  A. Symptoms noted on the Checklist include persistent neonatal vomiting, psychomotor retardation, sepsis, acidosis, hyperacusis, and intermittent ataxia.
  B. Neurological abnormalities to be noted include seizures, acute neurological problems, movement disorders, and progressive neurological damage.
  C. Another symptom might include historical comments regarding abnormal odors, such as the mousey odor of phenylketonuria or the sweet smell of the urine in maple syrup urine disease.
  D. Symptoms of a psychiatric disturbance may also indicate a metabolic disease.
  E. A history of a progressive disease course may also be useful in identifying such metabolic disorders as maple syrup urine disease, phenylketonuria, and hypothyroidism.

VII. Signs of a Possible Metabolic Disorder
  A. Failure to thrive, which is listed on the Metabolic Screening Checklist, is a nonspecific finding characteristic of many of the metabolic disorders; since failure to thrive that is not due to specific organic disease is nearly always due to a nutritional problem, the physician should ascertain whether the child is receiving adequate nutritional intake.
  B. Other signs include visceromegaly, abnormal dermatologic findings, abnormal facial features, ophthalmologic findings, and rachitic changes.
  C. If any signs and/or symptoms are noted, the physician should seek laboratory assistance in making a diagnosis; this should be done even if earlier routine screening yielded a negative result.

VIII. Laboratory Data
  A. A low pH and elevated anion gap suggest the need for a urine organic acid screen to investigate the possibility of unusual organic acid accumulation; hypoglycemia may be seen in a number of metabolic disorders.
  B. Bone marrow and peripheral blood tests may reveal stored material.
  C. Radiological findings of dysostosis multiplex are characteristic of certain storage diseases, as are degenerative changes in the ends of the long bones associated with central nervous system deterioration.

IX. Procedures for Ruling Out Metabolic Disorders
  A. To rule out metabolic disorders in all children who are suspected of being developmentally delayed, the physician should complete the Metabolic Screening Checklist and send it with blood and urine specimens to a regional metabolic laboratory.
  B. To assure that the laboratory knows what to do with the Checklist, it is suggested that the physician call the laboratory director and state the kind of assistance being sought.
  C. The Checklist seeks information which is important in interpreting blood and urine tests, including medication and diet.
  D. Because specific metabolic tests can be costly, the physician should try to arrange to have the state health department or a regional metabolic laboratory conduct the tests at minimal cost.

X. Case History
  A. The case involves a boy who was evaluated for failure to thrive at eight months, but whose phenylketonuria was not discovered until he was 26 months of age, at which time he functioned at the 10-month level.
  B. This case is one in which phenylketonuria screening failed to identify the condition; had the physician completed the Checklist recommended in this chapter at the eight month failure to thrive evaluation, the diagnosis would have been made then.

C. Had the primary care physician conducted routine developmental screening, the child would have been suspect before six months of age; in either case the phenylketonuria would have been discovered earlier and the child's prognosis would be better.

XI. Summary

INTRODUCTION

Inborn errors of metabolism were first described at the beginning of this century by Sir Archibald Garrod, a physician at University College Hospital in London. Individually they are rare diseases, but collectively they have attracted a great deal of interest because an increasing number of them can be treated successfully, and because their identification affords opportunities for genetic counseling. The combined prevalence of these disorders is estimated at one per 1,000 children.

To place this in perspective, consider an analogy to the polio epidemic of 1952, the last large epidemic prior to immunization. That year there were approximately 58,000 polio cases in the United States, or 367 cases per one million Americans. If the incidence of genetic metabolic disorders is one in 1,000, the extended frequency would be 1,000 per million population—a frequency three times that seen for polio during the 1952 epidemic year.

Without accurate diagnosis of metabolic disorders it is impossible to institute appropriate treatment. For some disorders, such as congenital hypothyroidism, which represents an inborn error or hormone biosynthesis, treatment consists of hormone supplementation. For conditions such as phenylketonuria, galactosemia, and maple syrup urine disease, where nonmetabolized substrates or toxic metabolites accumulate, treatment consists of putting the child on a special diet that is low in the particular substrate involved.

In the case of phenylketonuria, the body lacks the activity of a liver enzyme, phenylalanine hydroxylase, which is required to metabolize phenylalanine to tyrosine. Infants with phenylketonuria, therefore, accumulate excessive quantities of phenylalanine, which causes brain damage. Treatment consists of providing a phenylalanine-low milk substitute to prevent the excessive accumulation of phenylalanine in the body.

IMPORTANCE OF EARLY TREATMENT

Early treatment for metabolic disorders is necessary if mental retardation and other developmental problems are to be prevented or ameliorated.

For instance, appropriate treatment of maple syrup urine disease is essential within the first few weeks of life if life is to be sustained. Early treatment of galactosemia can reverse cataracts and prevent mental retardation. In the case of phenylketonuria, treatment begun within the first three weeks of life generally results in normal intellectual development; treatment delayed beyond the latter part of the first year usually results in irreparable mental retardation.

Similarly, the prognosis for intellectual development of infants with congenital hypothyroidism is directly related to the age at onset of treatment. The percentage of congenital hypothyroid patients eventually having I.Q.s of 85 and above is: 85 percent for those treated by three months of age; 25 percent for those treated by six months of age; and only 15 percent for those begun on treatment after six months of age.

As a way of illustration, consider the case of an infant with congenital hypothyroidism who was not identified until nine months of age. In retrospect, this child should have been identified much sooner in that he was an "ideal, good" baby who was passive and unresponsive. Originally, this was attributed to his two- to four-week prematurity. Developmentally he did not roll over until five months of age or hold his head erect until six months, and he was not sitting at nine months. At that age, the diagnosis became apparent and treatment was begun. Four months after treatment, his developmental evaluation was in the borderline retarded range with a developmental quotient of 69.

Only time will tell how this child will develop, but his prognosis would certainly have been far better if he had been identified with a neonatal thyroid screen or even a developmental screening test at three to four months.

Since development is a complex process—that is, influenced by a variety of biological and environmental factors—it is not surprising that exceptions to the above generalizations about prognosis are to be found. One of the most dramatic exceptions seen in the University of Colorado Metabolic Clinic was a phenylketonuric four-year-old child whose I.Q. was untestable; after beginning treatment, he rapidly became alert and responsive. When last seen, he had an I.Q. that was in the normal range. In view of these rare exceptions, it is important to identify children with metabolic disorders regardless of their age, and to determine if they will benefit from treatment.

The recognition of the importance of early treatment of these metabolic disorders and the development of simple, quick, and economical screening procedures have been the main reasons for the large-scale proliferation of neonatal screening for inborn errors of metabolism. Most states require screening for phenylketonuria, and many states also screen for hypothyroidism, maple syrup urine disease, and galactosemia.

The screening for congenital hypothyroidism is becoming more widespread as an ever-increasing number of professional groups, such as the American Academy of Pediatrics, recommend that such screening be made a routine procedure for all infants. The prevalence of this condition is estimated to be about one in 5,000 births. Articles pertaining to the screening for this disorder are listed in the attached bibliography.

One important fact should be remembered about metabolic screening—screening tests are not diagnostic. Screening will invariably fail to identify some children with metabolic disorders just as it will also err in generating false positive results. This point is particularly significant in the evaluation of a child who is suspected of being delayed in development, since the diagnosis of phenylketonuria has been delayed on more than one occasion because the physician conducting the evaluation has failed to recognize that false negative results do occur with screening. Such additional delays in diagnosis may produce irreparable handicaps.

Therefore, in evaluating a child who is suspected of delayed development, it is essential to rule out metabolic disorders through laboratory tests, even when previous screening tests for these conditions have been negative.

IMPLICATIONS FOR GENETIC COUNSELING

The importance of detecting metabolic disorders is not confined to identifying treatable conditions; another major reason for identifying such disorders is that there are implications for genetic counseling. This is especially important in a variety of metabolic diseases for which no treatment is presently available. Information from antenatal diagnosis offers women the option of not continuing a pregnancy when it would inevitably result in a severely damaged child. In other cases metabolic disorders can be diagnosed in the heterozygous state; then it is possible to counsel parents of options such as avoiding future pregnancies, adopting a child, or obtaining prenatal diagnosis.

The importance of such genetic counseling in the prevention of these metabolic disorders cannot be overemphasized when one considers the psychological grief and economic costs that have been spared in their prevention.

TABLE 9-1   Disorders of Protein Metabolism

1. Phenylketonuria		Rx	C
2. Maple Syrup Urine Disease	PD	Rx	
3. Homocystinuria	PD		
4. Cystinuria		Rx	C
5. Methylmalonic Aciduria	PD	Rx	

PD = Prenatal Dx available
Rx = Amenable to specific treatment
C = Carriers can be detected

TYPES OF METABOLIC DISORDERS

The three tables on this page provide a brief list of some of the most common inborn errors of metabolism encountered.

Table 9-1 is concerned with aminoacidopathies. Phenylketonuria is undoubtedly the most common and the most familiar on this list. Cystinuria is frequently associated with severe developmental retardation in children. Methylmalonic aciduria is of some technical interest because it has a very acute onset and because it requires certain rather sophisticated laboratory techniques for its prompt detection.

Table 9-2 lists some of the disorders of carbohydrate metabolism. Galactosemia is one disorder which presents acutely in the newborn period. Glycogen storage disease very often is present with hepatomegaly in young children.

Table 9-3 illustrates a group of diseases that have only recently been defined closely in terms of their actual enzyme deficiency. These are called the lysosomal storage diseases. Since many of them lead to very severe clinical handicaps, the importance of carrier detection and even more particularly for prenatal diagnosis is easy to see.

TABLE 9-2   Disorders of Carbohydrate Metabolism

1. Galactosemia	PD	Rx	C
2. Glycogen Storage Disease	PD	Rx	C
3. Mucopolysaccharidoses			
Hurler's Syndrome	PD		C
Sanfilippo Syndrome	PD		C

PD = Prenatal Dx available
Rx = Amenable to specific treatment
C = Carriers can be detected

TABLE 9-3   Lysosomal Storage Diseases

1. Tay-Sachs	PD	C
2. Nieman-Pick	PD	C
3. Gaucher's	PD	C
4. G_M Gangliosidosis	PD	C

PD = Prenatal Dx available
C = Carriers can be detected

IDENTIFICATION OF METABOLIC DISORDERS

To assist in the identification of metabolic disorders, a Metabolic Screening Checklist is included with this chapter as Appendix A.

First on the Checklist is the family history, which can be a diagnostic aid for the physician. Many families with a developmentally delayed child have a history of fetal wastage characteristic of the disorders of organic acid metabolism; common signs and symptoms of such disorders are metabolic acidosis and death. If siblings have had similar presentations and courses, this information can be helpful since many of these diseases are autosomal recessive. Other information which might be important in the family history would be knowledge of infant deaths, consanguinity, ethnic background, and other relatives with similar diseases. For example, the incidence of Tay-Sachs disease is increased significantly in Jews of Eastern European ancestry, as well as in certain French-Canadian subpopulations. Similarly, there seems to be a concentration of methylmalonic aciduria and possibly homocystinuria in the Mexican-American population.

SYMPTOMS WHICH INDICATE A POSSIBLE METABOLIC DISORDER

Each of the metabolic conditions which have been described is rare, and it would be extremely difficult for the physician to remember all of the symptoms. Instead, a patient manifesting any of the symptoms on the Checklist should be considered for the possibility of a metabolic disorder.

Persistent neonatal vomiting and

psychomotor retardation are symptoms of possible metabolic disease.

Symptoms of sepsis and acidosis are usually important in evaluating the critically ill newborn with a disturbance of amino acid or organic acid metabolism. For instance, a patient was recently diagnosed who had multiple episodes of a sepsis-like syndrome with acidosis, and who was found at approximately 18 months of age to have propionic acidemia. Similarly, a four-year-old girl with multiple episodes of acidosis and vomiting was ultimately diagnosed as having methylmalonic aciduria. In these cases, the vomiting probably represented a symptom of the recurring acidosis.

Hyperacusis and intermittent ataxia should also alert the physician to a possible metabolic disease. Intermittent ataxia may be seen with the hyperammonemias, Hartnup disease, and lactic acidemia. A movement disorder associated with basal ganglia disease and characterized by choreoathetosis may be found in glutaric acidemia, another of these rare disorders.

Neurological abnormalities include seizures with possible loss of consciousness. Phenylketonuria, for example, may cause seizures in the first six months of life. Acute neurological problems (such as convulsions), movement disorders (such as choreoathetosis), and progressive neurological damage are all listed on the Checklist.

Another symptom might include historical comments regarding abnormal odors, such as the mousey odor of the phenylketonuric or the sweet smell of the urine in maple syrup urine disease.

Symptoms of psychiatric disturbance may also indicate a metabolic disease and may be the reason for a developmental delay. For example, a pediatric neurologist recently saw a patient at the Colorado Psychiatric Institute for control of seizures. He noted this individual's Marfanoid habitus, and on the basis of an amino acid screen, made a diagnosis of homocystinuria. Similarly, some phenylketonuric patients manifest psychotic symptoms and are referred to psychiatric clinics where the diagnosis of phenylketonuria may not be considered.

A history of a progressive disease course may be useful in identifying metabolic disorders such as maple syrup urine disease, phenylketonuria, hypothyroidism, and so forth.

SIGNS OF A POSSIBLE METABOLIC DISORDER

The signs of special importance to note on physical examination are also listed on the Metabolic Screening Checklist.

The first is failure to thrive. This is a nonspecific finding characteristic of many of the metabolic disorders. Failure to thrive that is not due to specific organic disease is nearly always due to a nutritional problem. In evaluating this common clinical situation, it is particularly important for the physician to carefully ascertain if the child is receiving adequate nutritional intake.

Another sign is visceromegaly, which may be seen in many of the storage diseases.

Still another is abnormal dermatologic findings such as: the eczema of phenylketonuria; the underdevelopment of pigment, as seen in phenylketonuria or homocystinuria; or a history of prolonged jaundice, as may be seen with galactosemia.

Abnormal facial features may be characteristic of the mucopolysaccharidoses and certain other storage diseases.

Ophthalmologic findings that might be characteristic would be: the dislocated lens of the homocystinuric; the macular cherry red spot seen in Tay-Sachs disease and certain of the other storage diseases; and the corneal clouding of the patient with one of the mucopolysaccharidoses.

Rachitic changes, which could be thought of as indicating vitamin D deficiency, are more often seen in X-linked phosphaturic vitamin D resistant rickets or in Fanconi's syndrome with generalized amino aciduria and with numerous underlying etiologies including galactosemia, Wilson's disease, Lowe's oculo-renal-cerebral syndrome, and the syndromes of microcephaly and spastic diplegia.

If any of these signs and/or symptoms are observed, the physician should seek further support in making the diagnosis. Laboratory assistance should be sought even if earlier routine screening, as in the case of phenylketonuria, yielded a negative result.

LABORATORY DATA

Conventional laboratory data, if available, may be quite useful in the differential diagnosis of metabolic disorders. A low pH and elevated anion gap suggest the need for a urine organic acid screen to investigate the possibility of unusual organic acid accumulation. Hypoglycemia may be seen in a number of metabolic disorders including: hereditary fructose intolerance; galactosemia; other disorders of carbohydrate metabolism; maple syrup urine disease; methylmalonic acidemia; and other diseases of amino and organic acid metabolism.

Bone marrow as well as peripheral blood tests may reveal the stored material of many of the storage diseases. CSF protein is frequently elevated in metachromatic and Krabbe leucodystrophies.

Radiological findings of dysostosis multiplex (demonstrating the gibbus with breaking or hooking of the vertebral bodies, splaying of the distal ribs, broadened long bones, and shortened, thickened phalangeal bones) are characteristic of mucopolysaccharidoses and certain other storage diseases. Degenerative changes in the ends of the long bones associated with central nervous system deterioration are characteristic of juvenile Gaucher's disease.

PROCEDURES FOR RULING OUT METABOLIC DISORDERS

When evaluating children who are suspected of being delayed in development, it is essential that the physician rule out metabolic disorders. To do so, it is recommended that the physician complete the Metabolic Screening Checklist and send blood and urine specimens as instructed on the bottom of the Checklist to a regional metabolic laboratory. To assure that the laboratory knows what to do with the Checklist, it is suggested that the physician call the director of the laboratory to tell him or her the type of assistance being sought.

The Checklist seeks certain information which is important in terms of interpretation of the blood and urine tests. For example, it is useful to know if the patient is on any medication, since drugs may affect some of the screening tests. The information on the child's diet is requested for the same reason; specific formulas may result in unusual laboratory test results.

Blood and urine specimens will be utilized to perform routine tests of amino acid screening of blood and urine, and a TSH or T_4 determination to rule out hypothyroidism. Laboratory physicians will use the completed screening Checklist to consider what additional diagnostic tests should be performed; the Checklist responses may also suggest diagnoses to them that require additional specimens.

Because specific metabolic tests can be costly, the physician should try to make arrangements to have either the state health department or a regional metabolic laboratory conduct metabolic screening tests, for these entities frequently offer the tests at minimal cost. To locate the nearest diagnostic laboratory, the physician can contact the American Academy of Pediatrics.

CASE HISTORY

The following case history is provided for purposes of illustration. The patient, a Caucasian boy with a history of failure to thrive, was the 5-pound-4½-ounce product of a full-term uncomplicated gestation of a 17-year-old Gravida I Para I mother. The peri- and neonatal courses were uncomplicated. His early development was marked by delays in sitting, speech, and growth. At eights months of age the child was admitted to a hospital for a failure to thrive evaluation; after a multitude of tests, he was discharged with a primary diagnosis of caloric deprivation. At 26 months of age, he was referred for an evaluation of retarded development. A diagnosis of phenylketonuria was made on the basis of a serum phenylalanine of 37.0 milligrams per deciliter. At that time the boy functioned at the 10-month level with a development quotient of 39 (the normal being 100). Dietary treatment and a full-time special education program were begun promptly, and have been maintained to the present. The child's last three I.Q. scores, obtained when he was between five and seven years of age, averaged 60.

This case is one in which phenylketonuria screening failed to identify the condition. Even when the child was hospitalized at eight months for failure to thrive, the physician failed to test for phenylketonuria. As a result, the diagnosis was delayed until the child was 27 months of age, by which time the phenylketonuria had produced irreparable damage.

As part of the eight month work-up of failure to thrive, the physician following the protocol recommended in this chapter would have completed the Checklist as presented in Appendix B.

Had the physician submitted the blood and urine specimens, the report would have come back stating that the serum phenylalanine was markedly elevated (to 30 milligrams per deciliter), and that the physician should request serum tyrosine and check the urine for phenylpyruvic acid to substantiate the tentative diagnosis of phenylketonuria.

As has been seen, had the primary care physician conducted routine developmental screening, the child would have been suspect before six months of age. If the child had received the appropriate diagnostic evaluation at eight months (including the Metabolic Screening Checklist recommended in this chapter), phenylketonuria would have been detected far earlier, and the child's intellectual development would probably have been far better.

SUMMARY

The physician is not expected to remember all the signs and symptoms of the previously-named metabolic conditions. Instead, the physician should detect these disorders by filling out the enclosed Metabolic Screening Checklist and collecting blood and urine samples. Answers on the Checklist are of paramount importance to the physicians who will review the findings, formulate differential diagnoses, and who may recommend subsequent specific laboratory procedures to rule out some of the less common disorders.

To assure that cases of hypothyroidism and aminoacidopathies are not overlooked, blood and urine specimens should be collected according to the instructions on the bottom of the Checklist. Before sending the specimens and the Checklist, the physician should call the director of the regional laboratory to make him or her aware of specific requests.

Though metabolic diseases—even collectively—are extremely rare, they do occur with sufficient frequency to warrant consideration. For instance, one family practitioner in the small rural community of LaJunta, Colorado, was surprised to uncover two cases of phenylketonuria in his practice within the last five years.

In the consideration of metabolic disorders, the following points should be remembered whenever evaluating a child who manifests a developmental delay:

1. Any child manifests delays in development should be suspected of having an inborn error of metabolism regardless of what other causes are suspected.

2. Many of these disorders can be treated, and—in general—the earlier treatment is begun, the better the prognosis for the child.

3. Other disorders lend themselves to prenatal diagnosis and some to testing in the heterozygote state.

4. To avoid overlooking inborn errors of metabolism, the physician should complete the enclosed Checklist, send blood and urine specimens to the nearest regional metabolic laboratory, and call the director of the laboratory to explain specific requests.

APPENDIX A

Metabolic Screening Checklist

Name_____Hospital Number_____

Sex_____Age_____Age of Presenting Symptoms_____

Physician_____

   Address_____

Family History:

   Siblings with Fetal Wastage_____
   Siblings with Similar Retardation_____
   Infant Deaths (Sex and Age)_____
   Consanguinity_____Ethnic Background_____
   Relatives with Similar Diseases_____
   Other_____

Symptoms:

   Persistent Vomiting_____Ataxia_____
   Psychomotor Retardation_____Neurological Abnormalities_____
   Sepsis_____Acidosis_____
   Unusual Biological Fluid Odor_____Hyperacusis_____
   Psychiatric_____Other_____

Signs: (If positive, specify)

   Failure to Thrive_____Abnormal Facial Features_____
   Growth Percentiles: Head Circumference_____Height_____Weight_____
   Visceromegaly_____Abnormal Ophthalmic Findings_____
   Unusual Dermatologic Conditions_____Rachitic Changes_____

Course:

   Progressive_____Stable_____

Laboratory Data and Roentgenographic Findings:

   Serum pH_____Bone Marrow_____
   Bicarbonate_____CSF Protein_____
   Na_____K_____Cl_____X-rays_____
   Glucose_____Urinalysis_____
   Ketonuria_____Other_____

Medications Patient is Taking: _____

Nutrition:

   Breast Feeding_____Formula_____
   Indications of Nutritional Inadequacy_____
   Other_____

Differential Diagnosis: _____
_____

Specimen Requirements – to be sent with completed questionnaire to:

   Collect 1 ml of blood and allow to clot. Centrifuge and separate serum. Send
   0.2 – 0.5 ml of serum and 5 – 10 ml of urine (random sample; no preservatives).

RESULTS OF LABORATORY STUDIES
   Serum Amino Acids_____Urine Amino Acids_____
   TSH or T^4 (Normal is____for this age)_____
   Additional Specimen Requirements: _____
   _____

APPENDIX B

Metabolic Screening Checklist

Name _FRANK JOHNSTONE_____ Hospital Number_____

Sex _M_ Age _8 MOS._ Age of Presenting Symptoms _6 MONTH ONSET_____

Physician_____

  Address_____

Family History:

  Siblings with Fetal Wastage_____
  Siblings with Similar Retardation_____
  Infant Deaths (Sex and Age)_____
  Consanguinity_____ Ethnic Background _ANGLO_____
  Relatives with Similar Diseases_____
  Other_____

Symptoms:

  Persistent Vomiting_____✓____ Ataxia_____
  Psychomotor Retardation__✓____ Neurological Abnormalities _DELAYED NEURO. DEVELOP_
  Sepsis_____ Acidosis_____
  Unusual Biological Fluid Odor_____ Hyperacusis_____
  Psychiatric_____ Other_____

Signs: (If positive, specify)

  Failure to Thrive___✓_____ Abnormal Facial Features_____
  Growth Percentiles: Head Circumference _BELOW 3RD_% Height _10_% Weight _5TH_%
  Visceromegaly_____ Abnormal Ophthalmic Findings____
  Unusual Dermatologic Conditions _ECZEMA_____ Rachitic Changes_____

Course:

  Progressive_____ Stable__✓_____

Laboratory Data and Roentgenographic Findings:

  Serum pH_____ Bone Marrow_____
  Bicarbonate_____ CSF Protein_____
  Na____ K____ Cl____ X-rays_____ Urinalysis_____
  Glucose_____ Other_____
  Ketonuria_____

Medications Patient is Taking: _NONE_____

Nutrition:

  Breast Feeding __✓_____ Formula_____
  Indications of Nutritional Inadequacy _✓_____
  Other_____

Differential Diagnosis: _? DEVELOPMENT RETARDED; FAILURE TO THRIVE DUE TO LACK OF NUTRITIONAL INTAKE ?_

Specimen Requirements - to be sent with completed questionnaire to:

  Collect 1 ml of blood and allow to clot. Centrifuge and separate serum. Send
  0.2 - 0.5 ml of serum and 5 - 10 ml of urine (random sample; no preservatives).

RESULTS OF LABORATORY STUDIES

  Serum Amino Acids_____ Urine Amino Acids_____
  TSH or T^4 (Normal is _____ for this age)_____
  Additional Specimen Requirements: _____
  _____

BIBLIOGRAPHY

Fisher, D. A. Neonatal thyroid screening. *Pediatric Clinics of North America,* 1978, *25,* 423–430.

Scriver, C. R., and Rosenberg, L. E. *Amino acid metabolism and its disorders.* Philadelphia: W. B. Saunders Company, 1973.

Stanbury, J. B., Wyngaarden, J. B., and Frederickson, D. S. (Eds.). *The metabolic basis of inherited disease* (4th ed.). New York: McGraw-Hill, 1978.

Chapter 10

Goal

To develop skills in assessing children for genetic disorders and in referring families for genetic evaluation.

Objectives

At the end of this chapter, the physician should be able to:
- identify history significant in the genetic evaluation of a child;
- recognize congenital malformations when examining a child, and differentiate between these and a genetic disorder;
- explain the significance of major and minor congenital malformations;
- differentiate between the possible causes of developmental delay for children with congenital malformations and for those without congenital malformations;
- describe how and when to refer a family to a genetic counseling clinic.

GENETIC EVALUATION

By
EVA SUJANSKY, M.D.

I. Introduction
Genetic evaluation can help the physician counsel the parents of a handicapped child about future pregnancy risks, and can assist the physician in knowing when to refer a patient to a genetic counseling clinic.

II. Definition of Terms
  A. Congenital defects are those which are present at birth.
  B. Genetic disorders are those which cause defects through abnormal genes or chromosomes.
  C. Developmentally delayed children with congenital malformations do not necessarily have a genetic abnormality.

III. History-Taking
  A. A detailed family history should be taken.
  B. Past pregnancies of the parents should be investigated.
  C. A prenatal history should be obtained.
  D. Details of the delivery and neonatal period should be explored.
  E. Developmental milestones of the child should be obtained.

IV. Congenital Malformations
  A. Major malformations are those which affect the child's health and longevity.
  B. Minor malformations do not by themselves have clinical significance.

V. Physical Examination
Minor congenital malformations can be revealed through examination of the head and neck, chest and abdomen, extremities, and skin.

VI. Multiple Malformations
Major congenital defects and/or multiple minor malformations can indicate a chromosomal abnormality, an inherited single gene defect, a polygenically caused birth defect of CNS, nongenetic factors, or a syndrome of unknown etiology.

VII. Chromosomal Abnormalities
  A. New banding techniques of chromosome identification, which have identified a large number of different chromosomal abnormalities, are more accurate than previous techniques.
  B. Parents producing a child with a structural chromosomal abnormality may be at high risk for producing similarly affected children; chromosomal analysis is indicated on such parents to rule out a balanced chromosome translocation.
  C. If a balanced translocation is identified, parents should receive amniocentesis during subsequent pregnancies.
  D. All children with Down Syndrome should have chromosome analysis.
  E. If Down Syndrome is caused by translocation, one of the parents may be a balanced translocation carrier, in which case the mother should have prenatal diagnosis during subsequent pregnancies.

    F. If Down Syndrome is caused by simple trisomy 21, the parents may have an increased recurrence risk, and amniocentesis is indicated during subsequent pregnancies; the same applies to numerical abnormalities of other chromosomes.

    G. If a chromosome abnormality is suspected, the physician should send a sample of the patient's blood to a cytogenetic laboratory; if the result is positive, the family should be referred to a genetic counseling clinic.

VIII. Single Gene Defects

    A. Autosomal dominantly inherited diseases affect both sexes, may be present with different severity within the same family, and are vertically transmitted between generations; the recurrence risk for offspring of an affected parent is 50 percent.

    B. Autosomal recessive disorders affect siblings of normal parents; consanguinity between the parents makes this form of inheritance highly suspicious, and recurrence risk for siblings of an affected child is 25 percent.

    C. X-linked recessive inheritance usually only affects males, who are related to each other through unaffected females.

    D. If a single gene defect is suspected, the patient should be referred to a genetic counseling clinic.

    E. The affected child may represent a new mutation; then the recurrence risk for subsequent siblings is very low.

IX. Nongenetic Factors

    A. Irradiation can have a teratogenic effect on the fetus.

    B. Congenital infections such as rubella, toxoplasmosis, CMV, and herpes are known teratogens.

    C. Maternal alcoholism during the first trimester of pregnancy causes fetal alcohol syndrome in some exposed babies.

    D. Drugs such as dilantin, progestational agents, and anticoagulant coumadin, when taken during pregnancy, can cause birth defects.

    E. Maternal disease during pregnancy, including maternal phenylketonuria, can cause mental retardation.

X. Syndromes of Unknown Etiology

    A. Syndromes of unknown etiology usually occur sporadically.

    B. Such syndromes include Rubinstein-Taybi syndrome, and Elfin face or Williams syndrome.

XI. Absence of Congenital Malformations

Mental retardation in children without associated congenital malformations, such as familial, multifactorial mental retardation, may have a genetic basis.

XII. The Genetic/Birth Defect Screening Checklist

    A. The first portion of the Checklist, Summary of Present Findings, can be completed by an office assistant following completion of the history and of the physical and neurological examinations.

    B. The physician can use Part II, Suspected Etiology and Recommended Evaluation, to decide whether referrals are necessary.

    C. The Checklist can also serve as a brief case summary when a child is referred.

XIII. Genetic Counseling Referral

    A. Patients in whom it is impossible to establish an exact diagnosis should be referred for diagnostic work-up.

    B. If the physician is not familiar with a diagnosed disease, the patient should be referred for genetic counseling.

    C. Histories and all relevant information should be forwarded to the genetic counseling clinic prior to a family's first visit.

XIV. Summary

INTRODUCTION

The purposes of the following presentation are: (1) to help the physician determine which children with delayed development should be suspected of genetic disorders so that parents can be counseled as to the recurrence risk for future pregnancies; (2) to assist the physician in knowing which patients should be referred to a genetic counseling clinic; and (3) to provide information about what genetic counseling clinics offer patients.

DEFINITION OF TERMS

Children with developmental delays can be divided into two groups: those who have associated congenital malformations; and those without congenital malformations, in which the developmental delay is the only abnormality.

The term congenital defect means only that the defect is present at birth. It does not imply any genetic etiology. In contrast, genetic disorder means that the condition was caused by abnormal genes or chromosomes.

Some congenital disorders, such as Down Syndrome, are of genetic origin. Many congenital disorders, such as congenital rubella syndrome, are of nongenetic origin. This distinction is very important since it points out that developmentally delayed children with associated congenital malformations may, but do not have to, have a genetic abnormality; thus another etiology should be considered.

HISTORY-TAKING

The history can be of major significance in determining the etiology of the child's developmental delay, or can at least give clues to the etiology.

The physician should obtain information about the following areas:

1. A detailed family history should be taken, with close attention paid to possible clinical variability of a disease. The physician should search for possible symptoms in the patient's close relatives, and if necessary, perform a physical examination to detect mild symptoms.
2. Information should be collected on past pregnancies of the parents. If applicable, the history should include data about pregnancies from the parents' previous marriages. The physician should ask specifically about miscarriages, stillbirths, infertility, and births of abnormal children.
3. A detailed history of the pregnancy which resulted in the affected child should include possible maternal diseases and drugs used during the pregnancy.
4. Information should be compiled about the patient's labor, delivery, and neonatal period in search for a possible Rh incompatibility, oxygen deprivation, or intracranial injury.
5. Parents should be asked about the child's developmental milestones so the physician can assess the character of the developmental delay. The physician should determine if the early development was normal and then stopped, or if there has been continuous progress at a slower-than-normal rate.

CONGENITAL MALFORMATIONS

Congenital malformations found in children with developmental delays can be divided into two categories of clinical significance: major and minor malformations.

Major malformations are those which are significant for the patient's health and longevity. These include congenital heart disease, renal anomalies, meningomyelocele, cleft lip and palate, hydro- and microcephaly, and so forth, and certainly will not escape recognition.

Minor congenital malformations are those which do not by themselves have clinical significance. They may represent a cosmetic problem, or the patient and the family may not be concerned about them at all. These defects should be considered, however, since their presence in a mentally retarded child may indicate that the mental retardation was at least partially caused by a prenatal insult.

PHYSICAL EXAMINATION

Minor congenital malformations can be revealed during an examination of the head and neck, chest and abdomen, extremities, and skin.

The physician should examine the child's head for multiple hair whorls. Normally, one hair whorl occurs in the occipito-parietal area. Abnormal location of this whorl, or the presence of multiple hair whorls, may suggest abnormal development of the brain.

The physician should also look for symptoms of known hereditary syndromes. These include: sparce or breaking hair; a low, hairy forehead; abnormal eyebrows meeting at the midline (synophris); Mongoloid up-slanted occular fissues; antimongoloid down-slanted occular fissures; and hypertelorism (an increased distance between the eyes).

Other traits to look for around the eyes are epicanthal folds (abnormal folds at the inner aspect of the eyes), brushfield spots (grayish speckling of the iris), and short palpebral fissures.

The patient's nose may provide further clues; the physician should check for a depressed nasal bridge, a short, upturned nose and long philtrum, or a long, beaked nose and short piltrum. When examining the ears, the physician can look for abnormally shaped pinna and a narrow ear canal.

Coarse facial features may be indicative of storage disease. An abnormally shaped head may indicate premature closure of sutures. The neck may be short, may be webbed, or may have a redundant skin fold on the nape.

Examination of the chest may reveal shield chest, nipples set wide outside the mid-clavicular line, pectus excavatum, or mild scoliosis. The abdomen should be checked for umbilical hernia.

Malformations of the extremities include the following: asymmetry; hemihypertrophy; limbs disproportionately short or long in comparison to total body length; very long fingers (arachnodactyly) or fingers that are short and stubby; a

digitalised thumb; hypoplasia of fingernails and toenails; the Simian line (single transverse palmar crease as opposed to the normal two palmar creases); the Sydney line (the second palmar line extending across the whole palm); and increased distance between the first and second toes, or deep plantar furrow.

The skin should be examined for hypopigmented areas which may indicate tuberous sclerosis, or hyperpigmented lesions which may represent cafe au lait spots of neurofibromatosis. If present on the face, capillary hemangioma may indicate the presence of meningeal hemangioma.

MULTIPLE MALFORMATIONS

Although there are many other minor malformations, it would take too much space to discuss all of them here. However, the most important thing for the physician to remember is that any one minor malformation can be found in normal individuals. The presence of *more* of these minor malformations in a mentally retarded individual may be significant, as they may provide a clue for the diagnosis.

If a developmentally delayed child has one or more major congenital defects, multiple minor malformations, or a combination of minor and major defects, the following genetic etiologies should be considered:

1. a chromosomal abnormality;
2. a single gene defect inherited in an autosomal dominant, an autosomal recessive, or an X-linked recessive fashion;
3. a polygenically caused birth defect of CNS.

However, the condition could also be caused by *nongenetic* factors influencing intrauterine development, such as congenital infections and certain drugs; or it may represent a syndrome of unknown etiology.

CHROMOSOMAL ABNORMALITIES

In the 1970s new techniques were developed for chromosome identification.

The old technique enabled the identification of chromosomal abnormalities of a chromosomal number (such as Down Syndrome caused by trisomy 21, trisomy 13, or trisomy 18) or of very gross morphological changes such as a 13/21 translocation. However, more subtle chromosomal structural changes were missed by the old technique, because the difference in the size of a chromosome could be explained by the stretching or contracting of chromosomal material.

The new so-called "banding technique" produces light and dark stained bands across each chromosome which are identical for both members of a chromosomal pair; therefore, the absence or addition of a small portion of one chromosome can be identified by a missing band, or by the presence of an additional band.

Through this and other new techniques, approximately 100 different structural chromosomal abnormalities have been identified. Depending on the importance of the genes that normally occur on the portion of the chromosome which is missing or which is present in triplicate, more or less severe mental retardation or congenital malformations can result.

The identification of chromosomal abnormalities is important, even though it does not change the therapeutic approach to the patient. However, some couples having a child with a structural chromosomal abnormality may have a relatively high risk for having more children similarly affected. These couples should be identified, and prenatal chromosome analysis by utilizing amniocentesis should be offered to them.

One example is two boys, both with mental retardation and multiple minor morphologic anomalies (deep set eyes, short upturned noses, prognathia, and wide chests). These children were found to have additional chromosomal material on chromosome number 9. The pregnancy history of their mother was interesting in that, in addition to these two retarded sons, she had given birth to a stillborn baby with congenital malformations, and two other pregnancies had resulted in first trimester miscarriages.

When chromosome analysis was performed on the parents, the father's chromosomes were found to be normal. The mother had additional chromosomal material on chromosome number 9, like her two sons, but the same amount of material was missing on chromosome number 4. Therefore, she has what is called a "balanced chromosome translocation," and is normal. Her two abnormal sons have two whole chromosomes number 4 plus part of chromosome number 4 attached to chromosome number 9. They have an unbalanced chromosome translocation, and are therefore abnormal.

The mother, who later became pregnant, received prenatal diagnosis which documented that the chromosomes of the fetus were normal. This was confirmed by postnatal evaluation. If diagnosis of the chromosome abnormality had been made before the birth of her younger affected son, his birth could have been prevented.

For the same reason as is illustrated by this family, all children with a diagnosis of Down Syndrome should have chromosome analysis. Such an analysis can distinguish between those whose Down Syndrome is caused by simple trisomy 21, as opposed to those whose Down Syndrome is caused by translocation (where the third chromosome 21 is attached to another chromosome).

If the Down Syndrome is caused by translocation, there is increased risk that one of the parents is a balanced translocation carrier. This means that the parent has only one isolated chromosome 21, and that the second chromosome 21 is attached to another chromosome. This balanced translocation carrier, although not phenotypically abnormal, will be at increased risk for having more children with Down Syndrome. Therefore, other family members at risk of also having balanced translocation should be detected, and prenatal diagnosis should be offered to all balanced translocation carriers during all of their pregnancies.

The following case is from the University of Colorado Health Sciences Center's Genetic Counseling Clinic, and involves a family who came to the Clinic because their third child was born with Down Syndrome. The mother was 33 years old at that time. The parents had two normal children, and the family history was negative for both Down Syndrome and for miscarriages. Chromosome analysis of the affected baby revealed that he had a 14/21 translocation. His mother was a balanced translocation carrier, as were his maternal grandmother and his normal sister. All of his mother's siblings are now being analyzed for chromosome rearrangement to see whether any additional family members are at an increased risk for having a child with Down Syndrome.

To summarize, chromosomal abnormality is to be suspected in children with developmental delays and major congenital malformations. If a chromosome abnormality is suspected, the following options should be pursued:

1. The physician should obtain a sample of the patient's blood for chromosome analysis and send it to a cytogenetic laboratory.
2. The patient should be referred to a genetic counseling clinic.

SINGLE GENE DEFECTS

The second group of genetic disorders, single gene defects, can be inherited in an autosomal dominant, autosomal recessive, or X-linked recessive fashion.

Autosomal dominantly inherited diseases show a vertical transmission from generation to generation. They affect both sexes, and may be present with different severity in affected individuals in the same family. The absence of a positive family history does not rule out the presence of an autosomal dominant disorder, for the affected child may represent a new mutation. However, before the diagnosis of a new mutation is made, both parents must be carefully examined for mild symptoms of the disease. If the child truly represents a new mutation, the recurrence risk for the parents is close to zero; if one parent is affected, there is a 50 percent recurrence risk. Examples of autosomal dominant disorders are tuberous sclerosis and neurofibromatosis.

An autosomal recessive disorder is suspected if there is consanguinity between the patient's parents, or if two or more children of both sexes of normal parents are affected. Recurrence risk for the siblings of an affected child is 25 percent. An example of an autosomal recessive disorder is Smith-Lemli-Opitz syndrome. This syndrome is characterized by growth deficiency, ptosis of the eyelids, anteverted nostrils, hypospodias, cryptorchidism, and webbing between the toes. Another example is ataxia telangiectasia, which is characterized by ataxia and telangiectasias of such areas as the nose, buccal mucosa, or elsewhere.

The characteristic of X-linked recessive inheritance is that it usually only affects males who are related to each other through unaffected females. For example, Renpenning type mental retardation is a mild mental retardation in which affected males resemble normal family members. Since the affected males do not have any striking characteristic features, the diagnosis is made on the basis of compatible family history and by exclusion of other etiologic factors.

To repeat, single gene defects can be responsible for developmental delay in children with associated congenital malformation in cases where: (1) the distribution of individuals affected with the disorder in a family is compatible with AD, AR, or X-linked mode of inheritance; or, (2) a syndrome or disease known to be caused by a single gene defect can be diagnosed. An example of this sort of disorder is neurofibromatosis. If a single gene defect is suspected, the patient should be referred to a genetic counseling clinic for syndrome identification.

One additional fact should be noted. Polygenic congenital malformations of the central nervous system, such as meningomyelocele or structural abnormality of the brain, may be responsible for developmental delay in certain children.

NONGENETIC FACTORS

Agents which are known to cause or are suspected of causing mental retardation and congenital malformations by being teratogenic to the fetus include the following:

1. Irradiation can have a teratogenic effect on the fetus. Only therapeutic, high dose irradiation is known to be teratogenic, causing microcephaly, skeletal defects, and so forth.

2. Congenital infections such as rubella, toxoplasmosis, CMV, and herpes are known teratogens. Symptoms in some children include multiple congenital malformations, blindness, and mental retardation, while in other children the only symptom may be deafness. Evaluation for possible congenital infection should include skull X-ray for the presence of intracranial calcifications, and careful examination of the eye for possible chorioretinitis or cataracts. The diagnosis can be established by a positive viral culture from urine or nasopharynx, or by documentation of increasing antibody titers in the patient's serum. The material for these studies must be sent to a viral laboratory. If a congenital infection is responsible for the mental retardation, the recurrence risk for future children is low.

3. Drugs used by the mother during the first trimester of pregnancy can have a teratogenic effect on the fetus.
   (a) Chronic alcoholism of the mother during the first trimester of pregnancy causes fetal alcohol syndrome in some exposed babies. This syndrome is characterized by low birth weight, failure to thrive, and abnormal craniofacial features consisting of anteverted nostrils, depressed nasal bridge, low-set and malformed ears, short palpebral fissures, ptosis, and strabismus. Affected babies have a higher-than-normal incidence of congenital heart disease, microcephaly, and mental and motor retardation.
   (b) Dilantin during pregnancy may cause fetal hydantoin syndrome in 10 percent of exposed babies. This can consist of such major congenital malformations as cleft lip and/or palate, congenital heart disease, and microcephaly. Multiple minor malformations can include a short, upturned nose, hypertelorism, epicanthal folds, ptosis, low-set ears, wide mouth, hypoplastic distal phalanges, and hypoplastic fingernails and toenails.
   (c) Progestational agents in the form of birth control pills, provocation tests to diagnose pregnancy, or as treatment of a threatened abortion may cause a variety of congenital malformations. The combination of most frequent malformations is called the VACTERL syndrome (vertebral, anal, cardiac anomalies, T-E fistula, renal, and limb anomalies). The most common of these is congenital heart disease, incidence of which is two to three times increased in babies exposed to progestational agents during the first trimester of pregnancy.
   (d) Anticoagulant coumadin can cause craniofacial abnormalities, of which the most characteristic are nasal hypoplasia and X-ray finding of stippled epiphyses. Affected children may have mental retardation, optic atrophy, and cataracts.

4. The development of the fetus is also influenced by maternal diseases. One such disease is diabetes, which increases the frequency of congenital malformations. Another is maternal phenylketonuria. The physician must rule out maternal phenylketonuria, because a phenylketonuric mother who is not receiving treatment through a special diet will have high serum phenylalanine levels; these levels will cause mental retardation in practically 100 percent of offspring. The child of an untreated phenylketonuric mother will not him- or herself have phenylketonuria, as the child—although retarded—will have sufficient enzyme activity. Therefore maternal phenylketonuria should be ruled out in mothers of mentally retarded microcephalic infants. If the affected infant has normal older siblings, the physician can assume the absence of maternal phenylketonuria, since the presence of siblings with normal intelligence speaks against maternal phenylketonuria.

To review, the physician should be aware that children may have a developmental delay and congenital malformations if, during the first trimester of pregnancy, they are exposed to certain infections, drugs, therapeutic irradiation, or maternal diseases.

Detailed information about the pregnancy, including exposure to potential teratogens, should be obtained by the physician. Identification of teratogenic etiology is important for genetic counseling. Assuming that the teratogen would not be present during future pregnancies, the risk of recurrence is very low. The physician should not hesitate to contact a genetic clinic if there are questions about the teratogenicity of certain agents.

SYNDROMES OF UNKNOWN ETIOLOGY

Children may have congenital malformation and mental retardation caused by syndromes of unknown etiology. These syndromes usually occur sporadically.

Examples of such syndromes are as follows:

1. Rubinstein-Taybi syndrome is characterized by slow growth. The typical Rubinstein-Taybi syndrome child has a beaked nose, an antimongoloid slant of the eyes, abnormally wide angulated thumbs, and wide toes.
2. Elfin face or Williams syndrome is characterized by an elfin face, mental retardation, and a cardiovascular anomaly (mainly supravolvular aortic stenosis). Hypercalcemia may be detected during the first year of life.

ABSENCE OF CONGENITAL MALFORMATION

The second group of children with developmental delays are those without associated congenital malformations. Mental retardation in these children may also have a genetic basis. Each child inherits from the parents a large number of genes which influence the child's intelligence. The combination of genes which the child obtained, in addition to environmental factors, determines the child's intellectual capacity.

The child with familial mental retardation will have mild mental retardation. The intelligence of the patient's parents and siblings will be on a similar level, and the child will not have congenital malformations, since the mental retardation was not caused by a specific major insult. Of course, the diagnosis of familial mental retardation has to be made by the exclusion of such other etiologic factors as those which were discussed previously.

Some children without associated congenital malformations will be developmentally delayed or mentally retarded, although no etiological factors will be determined. Hence, the etiology will remain unknown.

THE GENETIC/BIRTH DEFECT SCREENING CHECKLIST

Because the material presented in this chapter is complex, a Genetic/Birth Defect Screening Checklist has been included as Appendix A. Part I of the Checklist, Summary of Present Findings, can be completed by a nurse or skilled office assistant following completion of the history and of the physical and neurological examinations.

The physician can then, in a minimum amount of time, use Part II of the Checklist, Suspected Etiology and Recommended Evaluation, to determine whether action must be taken in the case of a suspect child. The Checklist is designed not only to remind the physician when to order chromosomal studies and when to refer to a genetic counseling clinic; in addition, it can serve as a brief case summary when a child is referred. (Appendix B, a Checklist partially completed as if by an office assistant, is included to provide practice in the use of the Checklist.)

GENETIC COUNSELING REFERRAL

Guidelines for referring a child to a genetic clinic are listed below:

1. Patients in whom it is impossible to establish an exact diagnosis should be referred for diagnostic work-up, including a chromosome or other study if indicated.
2. If an exact diagnosis is possible but the physician is not familiar enough with all aspects of the disease, the child and his or her family may be referred to a genetic clinic.

A genetic clinic can answer questions for the family about the prognosis for the affected child, symptoms of the disease, the risk for the family of having a similarly affected child, the availability of a carrier test to identify family members at risk, the effectiveness of prenatal diagnosis, and the alternatives available for the parents to avoid having more affected children.

When the physician refers a child to a genetic clinic, all previously-mentioned information should be forwarded to clinic personnel prior to the patient's first visit. That information should include results of previous lab tests.

When an evaluation is completed, most genetic counseling clinics send a summary letter to the family and to the referring physician.

SUMMARY

In reviewing a child from a genetic standpoint, the physician should first take a history. Particular emphasis should be placed on the family history, the mother's pregnancy history, and the prenatal and perinatal history of the presenting child. The physician should assess the child for congenital malformations. If possible, the physician should also try to determine the etiology of the child's delay or retardation. The physician may decide that it is best to refer the family to a genetic counseling clinic.

As previously mentioned, the purpose of this presentation was not to explain methods of recognizing specific genetic disorders. Of course, physicians interested in this area may attempt to identify a specific syndrome by comparing the patient's abnormalities with syndromes described in available literature. However, this chapter was designed to provide background information on the characteristic features of conditions which are known to be inherited. These conditions should be recognized as such, since the family should be made aware of their recurrence risk. Recognition of known syndromes which are not genetic is equally valuable, because the family can be counseled that they have a low recurrence risk. There have been too many families who, following the birth of a mentally retarded child, feared to have more children because they were not given reasonable reassurances.

APPENDIX A

Genetic/Birth Defect Screening Checklist

Name of Child_____

Birthdate_____Date_____

I. Summary of Present Findings

    A. History

        1. Family History (close relatives with congenital abnormalities, such as mental retardation, multiple miscarriages, consanguinity): _____

            _____

            _____

        2. Past Pregnancy History (include information from previous marriages):

            Miscarriages_____Stillbirths_____

            Infertility_____Birth defects_____

        3. Pregnancy History (specify trimester):

            Irradiation_____Maternal illness_____

            Drugs_____Bleeding_____

            Birth control pills_____Alcohol_____

        4. Delivery and Neonatal History:

            Rh incompatability_____Intrauterine growth retardation_____

            Intracranial injury_____Other_____

        5. Developmental History (include whether development was initially normal and cite specific landmarks):

            _____

            _____

            _____

    B. Medical Examination

        1. Major Congenital Abnormalities (affecting major body organs):

            _____

            _____

            _____

        2. Minor Congenital Abnormalities (see items marked with * on Physical Examination form):

            _____

            _____

            _____

II. Suspected Etiology and Recommended Evaluation

    A. Chromosomal Abnormality

        1. Suspect a chromosomal abnormality if either:

            a. Child is developmentally delayed and has a major congenital abnormality; or

            b. Child is developmentally delayed and has two or more minor congenital abnormalities.

2. Disposition of suspected chromosomal abnormality:

   a. Refer for chromosome analysis;

   b. Refer to a genetic counseling clinic, accompanying referral with this completed Checklist and results of all previous laboratory tests.

B. Teratogenic Agent

  1. Non-TORCH

    a. Suspect a non-TORCH teratogenic agent if the following are noted under History and/or Medical Examination:

Maternal irradiation_____Maternal medications*_____

Maternal alcoholism_____Chronic maternal disease_____

Intrauterine growth retardation_____

Major and/or minor malformations_____

    b. Disposition if suspect non-TORCH teratogenic etiology:

Counsel parents of low recurrence risk if teratogenic agent will not be present in future pregnancies.

If in doubt as to diagnosis, refer to a genetic clinic. Accompany referral with this completed Checklist and results of all previous laboratory tests.

  2. TORCH

    a. Suspect a congenital TORCH infection (TOxoplasmosis, Rubella, Cyto-megalovirus, Herpes Simplex) if one or more of the following are present:

Abortions, stillbirths_____Lethargy, poor feeding_____

Prematurity, intrauterine growth retardation_____

Hepatosplenomegaly, jaundice_____Anemia_____

Petechiae, ecchymosis_____Congenital heart disease_____

Myocarditis, pneumonitis_____Encephalitis_____

Microcephaly_____Hydrocephalus_____

Intracranial calcification_____Hearing loss_____

Chorioretinitis_____Visual impairment_____

    b. Disposition if suspect TORCH:

Obtain antibody titers in neonatal and postnatal periods to demonstrate a rise in titer. (A single elevated viral titer and/or isolation of a virus do not establish an etiological agent in most cases, since the virus may be perinatally or postnatally acquired. A single titer may be virtually diagnostic in the case of rubella within the first 12 to 18 months if the child has not been immunized for rubella.) Whenever TORCH is suspected and antibody titers are obtained, a VDRL should also be ordered to rule out congenital syphilis.

For the older child suspected of having a congenital infection with TORCH on the basis of the signs and symptoms listed above, consultation may be sought from a pediatrician who specializes in the diagnosis and treatment of infectious diseases.

*If uncertain about teratogenicity of medications, check with a genetic center.

C. Single Gene Defect

    1. Suspect a single gene defect if chromosome studies and teratogenic evaluations are negative, and one of the two following points applies:

        a. The child is developmentally delayed and manifests one or more major anomalies; or

        b. The child is developmentally delayed and manifests two or more minor anomalies.

    2. Disposition if a single gene defect is suspected but a specific genetic disorder cannot be identified:

        Refer to a genetic clinic, accompanying the referral with a copy of the completed Genetic/Birth Defect Checklist and results of all previous laboratory tests.

APPENDIX B

Genetic/Birth Defect Screening Checklist

Name of Child *MARIA G.*

Birthdate *(CURRENTLY 2 YRS, 9 MONTHS)* Date _____

I. Summary of Present Findings

    A. History

        1. Family History (close relatives with congenital abnormalities, such as mental retardation, multiple miscarriages, consanguinity): *MOTHER'S BROTHER DIED AT 5 MONTHS OF CONGENITAL HEART DISEASE. MATERNAL SECOND COUSIN BORN WITH AORTIC VALVE STENOSIS. FATHER'S BROTHER DIED EARLY INFANCY, CAUSE UNKNOWN.*

        2. Past Pregnancy History (include information from previous marriages):

           Miscarriages _____ Stillbirths _____

           Infertility _____ Birth defects _____

        3. Pregnancy History (specify trimester):

           Irradiation _____ Maternal illness *NAUSEA AND VOMITING IN FIRST 5 MONTHS*

           Drugs _____ Bleeding _____

           Birth control pills _____ Alcohol _____

        4. Delivery and Neonatal History:

           Rh incompatability _____ Intrauterine growth retardation _____

           Intracranial injury _____ Other *VSD AND PULMONARY ATRESIA AT BIRTH; AORTO-PULMONARY ARTERY ANASTOMOSIS PERFORMED AT 2 DAYS*

        5. Developmental History (include whether development was initially normal and cite specific landmarks): *MOTOR DEVELOPMENT DELAYED FROM 2 MOS. CURRENTLY CANNOT WALK ALONE, PULL TO STAND, OR CRAWL. CAN ROLL OVER, & SIT & WALK IN A WALKER. CANNOT FEED SELF. HAS ONLY 3-4 WORDS. FAILURE TO THRIVE NOTED AT 2 MOS; CURRENTLY IS LESS THAN 3% BY WEIGHT AND HEIGHT.*

    B. Medical Examination

        1. Major Congenital Abnormalities (affecting major body organs): *CONGENITAL HEART DISEASE*

        2. Minor Congenital Abnormalities (see items marked with * on Physical Examination form): *FISTULA AT TIP OF NOSE, SIMIAN LINES, LOW-SET EARS, NARROW EAR CANALS, FIFTH FINGERS CURVE IN, HYPERTELORISM*

II. Suspected Etiology and Recommended Evaluation

    A. Chromosomal Abnormality

        1. Suspect a chromosomal abnormality if either:

           a. Child is developmentally delayed and has a major congenital abnormality; or

           b. Child is developmentally delayed and has two or more minor congenital abnormalities.

   2. Disposition of suspected chromosomal abnormality:

     a. Refer for chromosome analysis;

     b. Refer to a genetic counseling clinic, accompanying referral with this completed Checklist and results of all previous laboratory tests.

B. Teratogenic Agent

   1. Non-TORCH

     a. Suspect a non-TORCH teratogenic agent if the following are noted under History and/or Medical Examination:

Maternal irradiation_____Maternal medications*_____

Maternal alcoholism_____Chronic maternal disease_____

Intrauterine growth retardation_____

Major and/or minor malformations_____

     b. Disposition if suspect non-TORCH teratogenic etiology:

Counsel parents of low recurrence risk if teratogenic agent will not be present in future pregnancies.

If in doubt as to diagnosis, refer to a genetic clinic. Accompany referral with this completed Checklist and results of all previous laboratory tests.

   2. TORCH

     a. Suspect a congenital TORCH infection (TOxoplasmosis, Rubella, Cytomegalovirus, Herpes Simplex) if one or more of the following are present:

Abortions, stillbirths_____Lethargy, poor feeding_____

Prematurity, intrauterine growth retardation_____

Hepatosplenomegaly, jaundice_____Anemia_____

Petechiae, ecchymosis_____Congenital heart disease_____

Myocarditis, pneumonitis_____Encephalitis_____

Microcephaly_____Hydrocephalus_____

Intracranial calcification_____Hearing loss_____

Chorioretinitis_____Visual impairment_____

     b. Disposition if suspect TORCH:

Obtain antibody titers in neonatal and postnatal periods to demonstrate a rise in titer. (A single elevated viral titer and/or isolation of a virus do not establish an etiological agent in most cases, since the virus may be perinatally or postnatally acquired. A single titer may be virtually diagnostic in the case of rubella within the first 12 to 18 months if the child has not been immunized for rubella.) Whenever TORCH is suspected and antibody titers are obtained, a VDRL should also be ordered to rule out congenital syphilis.

For the older child suspected of having a congenital infection with TORCH on the basis of the signs and symptoms listed above, consultation may be sought from a pediatrician who specializes in the diagnosis and treatment of infectious diseases.

*If uncertain about teratogenicity of medications, check with a genetic center.

C. Single Gene Defect

   1. Suspect a single gene defect if chromosome studies and teratogenic evaluations are negative, and one of the two following points applies:

      a. The child is developmentally delayed and manifests one or more major anomalies; or

      b. The child is developmentally delayed and manifests two or more minor anomalies.

   2. Disposition if a single gene defect is suspected but a specific genetic disorder cannot be identified:

     Refer to a genetic clinic, accompanying the referral with a copy of the completed Genetic/Birth Defect Checklist and results of all previous laboratory tests.

BIBLIOGRAPHY

Clarren, S. K., and Smith, D. W. The fetal alcohol syndrome. *New England Journal of Medicine,* 1978, *298,* 1063–1067.

deGrouchy, J., and Tureau, C. *Clinical atlas of human chromosomes.* New York: John Wiley and Sons, 1977.

Hanson, J. W. Risk to the offspring of women treated with hydantoin anticonvulsants, with emphasis on the fetal hydantoin syndrome. *Journal of Pediatrics,* 1976, *89,* 662–668.

Hardy, J. B. Immediate and long-range effects of maternal viral infection in pregnancy birth defects. *Original Article Series,* 1976, *12* (5), 23–31.

Lubs, M. L. E., and Maes, J. A. Recurrence risk in mental retardation. In P. Mittler (Ed.), *Research to practice in mental retardation: Biomedical aspects* (Vol. 3). Baltimore: University Park Press, 1977.

Milunsky, A. *The prevention of genetic disease and mental retardation.* Philadelphia: W. B. Saunders Company, 1975.

Smith, D. *Recognizable patterns of human malformation.* Philadelphia: W. B. Saunders Company, 1976.

Chapter 11

Goal   To develop an awareness of the role of the psychologist in evaluating children suspected of developmental delay.

Objectives   At the end of this chapter, the physician should be able to:
- state the difference between screening and psychological tests;
- explain the kinds of cognitive and emotional assessments which a child psychologist can make;
- discuss autistic-like behavior and why an accurate diagnosis of children with this behavior is important;
- locate a qualified psychologist;
- discuss information which the physician should provide on referral.

PSYCHOLOGICAL EVALUATION

By
GORDON ULREY, Ph.D.

I. Introduction
Psychological tests, when administered by a trained psychologist, can help the primary care physician diagnose a developmental delay.

II. Differences Between Screening and Psychological Tests
   A. Some physicians suspecting a developmental delay use a screening test to confirm their diagnosis; they believe that screening tests negate the need for psychological testing.
   B. Because screening tests are not diagnostic and generate errors in both over- and underreferrals, they should not be substituted for psychological testing.

III. Overview of the Psychological Evaluation
   A. The psychologist first takes a history to determine what specific issues to consider, since there is no standard test or battery of tests given to every child.
   B. The physician must give the psychologist the specific concern or concerns that initiated referral.

IV. Infant Testing
   A. Tests used with infants and nonverbal children are substantially different from those used with older, verbal children.
   B. Infant tests, such as the Bayley Scales of Infant Development, provide an in-depth picture of a child's developmental status and psychomotor skills; many also permit observation of mother-child interactions.
   C. A major issue with infant tests is that they require a psychologist skillful in working with very young children.

V. Preschool Testing
   A. Tests used for children between two and six years of age include the Stanford-Binet Intelligence Scale, the Wechsler Preschool and Primary Scale of Intelligence, and the McCarthy Scales of Children's Abilities.
   B. Intelligence tests measure a variety of verbal and nonverbal skills, and can estimate a child's ability or intelligence.
   C. Because a nonverbal measure of intelligence is not as predictive as verbal skills, psychologists generally avoid reporting I.Q. scores for children under age six.

VI. Additional Psychological Assessments
   A. During an assessment the psychologist can observe the child's: ability to maintain attention; strategies in problem-solving; reactions to success or failure; methods of relating to strange adults; and learning style.
   B. An additional observation is of the parent-child relationship.

VII. Emotional/Behavioral Evaluation
   A. A physician who is concerned about a child's behavior can request an in-depth psychological evaluation of the child's emotional status.

    B. The psychologist, in addition to conducting psychological test-ing, will observe the child's behavior in a less structured setting.
    C. The psychologist will attempt to determine the extent to which emotional problems affect a developmental delay, and the extent to which a developmental delay has affected emotional development.

VIII. Autistic-Like Behavior
    A. Although true autism is extremely rare, the physician may recognize some of the signs and symptoms of autism in the behavior of suspect children.
    B. These signs and symptoms include difficulty in relating to people, lack of eye contact, failure to show affection, and repetitive activities.
    C. An accurate diagnosis is important because there are implica-tions for the child's treatment and prognosis.
    D. The psychologist is trained to help the physician decide when evaluation or treatment by a psychiatrist is necessary.

IX. Locating a Qualified Psychologist
    A. To locate a qualified child psychologist, the physician can:
       1. Ask the State Board of Psychological Examiners;
       2. Call the nearest mental health center;
       3. Ask a colleague to recommend a qualified psychologist.
    B. Once a psychologist has been located, the physician should describe the child's problem and ask if the psychologist tests young children; the physician should also ask the name of a psychiatrist who would be recommended for further referal, should that be necessary.
    C. If a child is suspected of multiple handicaps, referral can be made to a large medical center for an interdisciplinary evaluation.

X. Information to Supply on Referral
On referral, the physician should provide information about:
    1. The child's impairment;
    2. Significant elements in the history;
    3. Medications which could affect behavior;
    4. The precise concern for which the child is being referred.

XI. Parental Responses
    A. It may be necessary for the physician to play an active role in getting the parents to follow through on referral to a psychologist.
    B. The physician will probably want to discuss with the psychologist how results should be reported to parents.
    C. Most psychologists will prefer to be involved with interpreting findings to parents and helping them work through emotional reactions.

XII. Summary

INTRODUCTION

Psychological tests, when adminis-tered by a trained psychologist, can help the primary care physician diagnose a de-velopmental delay. Some general ques-tions that a psychologist using these tests can answer include the following:

1. Is there significant delay of cognitive and/or social-emotional development, and if so, to what degree?

2. Does the child show general develop-mental delay or specific disabilities, and what are the child's strengths and weaknesses?

3. Are the child's problems primarily a function of intellectual deficits or are they caused by emotional disorders stemming from familial or other rela-tionships or experiences?

DIFFERENCES BETWEEN SCREENING AND PSYCHOLOGICAL TESTS

Before discussion of how a psychological evaluation can be useful to the primary care physician, one important point should be considered. Some physicians who suspect a child in their practice of a developmental delay tend to administer a screening test—such as the Denver Developmental Screening Test (DDST)—to confirm that problem. These physicians feel that a screening test negates the need for psychological testing.

Nothing could be further from correct. Screening tests are very useful in identifying suspect children in an apparently well population, but as has been stressed earlier in the chapter on developmental screening, screening tests are *not* diagnostic. While screening tests can help identify a suspect child, they do not diagnose the child's delay. In addition, most screening tests generate some errors in both over- and underreferrals. Thus, if the physician suspects a child of a delay and attempts to make a diagnosis by using a screening test such as the DDST, the result may be very misleading; the screening test may generate a negative result when the child actually *has* the problem which is suspected. For these reasons, the physician should use screening tests for the purpose for which they were created—for screening—*not* for diagnosis.

OVERVIEW OF THE PSYCHOLOGICAL EVALUATION

When conducting a psychological evaluation, the psychologist first takes a history to determine what specific issues to address; the psychologist also considers the physician's specific referral questions. Since there is no standard test or battery of tests given to every child referred for psychological evaluation, the testing procedures a psychologist uses depends in part on what questions the physician asks. For this reason, the psychologist must be given the specific concern or concerns that initiated referral. For example, when a parent is concerned about overac-

tivity and how to manage behavior, there is little need for formal testing; the psychologist may rely more on family history and observations of the parent and child together in settings with different amounts of structure. The child's problems are always assessed in the context of the family. When there is concern about the degree of a child's delay, standardized tests are useful. When a child's disability is already identified, the referral question may focus on what can be done to encourage intellectual growth. In such latter cases, the psychologist may use tests that measure specific skill areas which emerge sequentially, to determine both what the child is able to do and what subsequent skills can be expected to develop.

INFANT TESTING

Table 11–1 provides an overview of infant tests, including the ages for which they are useful, what they measure, and their strengths and limitations. As might be imagined, the tests used with infants and nonverbal children are substantially different from those used with older, verbal children.

One test frequently used with very young children and/or very delayed children is the Bayley Scales of Infant Development. The Bayley measures a child's awareness and ability to act on what is perceived—in short, it measures general psychomotor skills. In addition to measuring these skills, it gives the psychologist administering the Bayley an opportunity to observe mother-child interactions. Infant tests such as the Bayley provide an in-depth picture of a child's current developmental status and psychomotor skills. This information is valuable for diagnosis of children with significant learning handicaps. These tests have some limitations. For example, they do not predict later intellectual development of normal children; however, significant delays on these tests are predictive of later disabilities.

One major issue with the infant tests is that they require a psychologist who is skillful in working with very young children. Since infants are easily distracted,

TABLE 11-1 Major Cognitive Tests for Young Children

Test	Ages Covered	Areas Measured	Strengths	Weaknesses
Bayley Scales of Infant Development: Mental Scale	2–30 months	Level of sensorimotor skills; problem-solving skills; measurements of verbal and nonverbal skills	Comprehensive developmental picture of child; indicates degree of developmental delay and reflects strengths and weaknesses of individual child	Does not predict later I.Q. or school performance unless child has significant delay of skills
Cattell Infant Intelligence Scale	2–30 months	Same as Bayley	Individual specific age levels and degrees of delayed development; a downward extension of the Stanford-Binet	Fewer items than Bayley; is based on a limited number of subjects
Merrill-Palmer Scales	1½–6 years	General intelligence; can be used as a non-verbal test; yields a mental age equivalency	Useful with language delayed and/or overactive children	Scores do not predict later school performance; predominance of nonverbal items
Leiter International Performance Scale	2–9 years	Nonverbal intelligence; items are mostly perceptual problem-solving	Used with hearing impaired, language delayed and motor handicapped children	Measures a minor range of intellectual skills; therefore limits description of child's strengths and weaknesses
Stanford-Binet Intelligence Scale	2 years–adult	General intelligence; cognitive strengths and weaknesses in both verbal and non-verbal skills	Best available test for prediction of school learning problems	Requires normal sensory and motor skills for valid results; predominance of verbal items
Wechsler Preschool and Primary Scale of Intelligence	4–6½ years	Verbal performance and full-scale intelligence	Yields profile of child's strengths and weaknesses on a wide range of skills	Limited age range; limited prediction of school learning problems
McCarthy Scales of Children's Abilities	2½–8½ years	General cognitive index and six areas of verbal and nonverbal skills	Provides an assessment of verbal and nonverbal skills	Difficult for child with developmental delays to complete; requires good attending and verbal skills

the examiner must elicit responses carefully for results to be valid. In addition, the psychologist must determine if sensory or motor problems have influenced the outcome.

PRESCHOOL TESTING

The preschool child is able to perform more advanced tasks, including verbal items. The Stanford-Binet Intelligence Scale is one of the best tests of general intellectual ability for use with children between the ages of two and six. Two other well-known tests are the Wechsler Preschool and Primary Scale of Intelligence, and the McCarthy Scales of Children's Abilities. These are also listed in Table 11–1.

Intelligence tests measure a variety of verbal and nonverbal skills which can be used to estimate a child's ability or intelligence. However, not all skills at an early age are predictive of later skill development. For example, a nonverbal measure of intelligence is not as predictive as are verbal skills. For this reason, psychologists generally avoid reporting I.Q. scores with children under six years of age because they are often not predictive of future performance and are an oversimplification of the child's strengths and weaknesses in cognitive areas.

ADDITIONAL PSYCHOLOGICAL ASSESSMENTS

In addition to test scores, the psychologist can provide other useful information. For example, during a psychological evaluation the psychologist can observe:

1. the child's ability to maintain attention, which relates to questions of hyperactivity;
2. the strategies the child uses in problem-solving, which helps reveal the child's level of intelligence;
3. the child's reactions to success or failure, which relate to environmental factors and/or learning deficits;
4. the way the child relates to a strange adult, which gives clues to emotional maturity; and
5. the child's learning style, which has implications for the need for early intervention and which can suggest the best approach to teaching.

One additional observation a psychologist makes during developmental testing is of the parent-child relationship. This observation can help reveal whether or not the parents are meeting the child's physical and emotional needs, and has obvious importance to both the physician's diagnosis and treatment plan.

EMOTIONAL/BEHAVIORAL EVALUATION

It has been noted that during developmental testing psychologists routinely make observations of a child's emotional and behavioral development. However, if the physician is concerned that the child's behavior is abnormal, he or she may wish to ask the psychologist for an in-depth evaluation of the child's emotional status.

Some examples of behavior which might indicate that an emotional assessment is needed include the following:

1. a child whose attachment to its mother seems either excessive or lacking;
2. a child with extreme difficulty relating to other people;
3. a child whose behavior seems to be interfering with the mastery of developmental tasks; and
4. a child whose affective behavior is of concern—for example, a child who is abnormally sad, shy, anxious, angry, withdrawn, and so on.

If the physician or the parents are concerned about a child's behavior, the psychologist should specifically be asked for an emotional assessment of that child. In addition to conducting developmental testing, the psychologist will observe the child's behavior in less structured settings. For example, the psychologist may first observe the child alone in a playroom, and then may observe as the mother and child interact in that room. Through such observations the psychologist will attempt to determine the extent to which emotional problems are affecting the child's behavior, and the effect that a developmental delay may have on emotional development—as well as the effect that emotional problems may have on a developmental delay.

AUTISTIC-LIKE BEHAVIOR

One behavioral problem which deserves additional attention is autistic-like behavior. Autism will be discussed because physicians who see children with behavior problems frequently believe these children are autistic.

True autism is extremely rare. Obviously the primary care physician is not expected to diagnose autism, for making such a diagnosis requires specialized training. Nevertheless, the physician may recognize some of the signs and symptoms of autism in the behavior of children suspected of developmental delay. For instance, the child may have trouble in relating to people as manifested by delayed language development, lack of eye contact, and failure to show affection. Such children may also have a preoccupation with repetitive activity such as spinning wastebaskets, ashtrays, or other miscellaneous objects, or with flicking light switches for long periods of time. The cause (or causes) of autism is not yet known. Some researchers suspect that it is due to impaired neurological function. This would explain why so many retarded and neurologically impaired children display some of the autistic-like behaviors mentioned.

A physician who sees children manifesting such behavioral characteristics should mention that fact to the psychologist to whom he or she is referring. An accurate diagnosis is important, for there are implications for treatment of the child and for the child's eventual prognosis depending on whether the child is truly autistic or (as is more common) retarded—or both.

A psychologist examining a child with behavior difficulties or autistic-like behavior patterns may feel confident that the child can be competently treated and the family counseled by a physician-psychologist team. However, there may be other times when the physician or the psychologist believe that psychoactive medications—which are probably best prescribed by a psychiatrist—are needed to manage a severely disturbed child. Part of a psychologist's training is to know when to refer for clinical services, including when to recommend that the physician refer a child to a psychiatrist. Thus the primary care physician does not have to be concerned about determining alone when to refer a child with a behavior problem for psychiatric assistance; the psychologist is trained to help make that determination.

LOCATING A QUALIFIED PSYCHOLOGIST

It is not always easy to locate an acceptable psychologist, since surprisingly few clinical psychologists have training and experience with very young children. Obviously in rural areas the difficulties may be increased. If an experienced child psychologist is not available, compromises may have to be made. For example, if a psychologist trained in evaluating a child's emotional status is not available, the physician may have to refer to a school psychologist whose training is largely in the area of cognitive evaluations. Similarly, it may be necessary to refer to a social worker, although a social worker normally concentrates more on counseling families than conducting psychological evaluations.

Some general guidelines to help locate a qualified psychologist include the following:

1. ask the State Board of Psychological Examiners for the names of licensed people;
2. call the nearest mental health center and ask advice on the best local resource;
3. ask a colleague to recommend a child psychologist.

Once a psychologist has been located, the physician should describe his or her concern and ask if the psychologist tests infants and preschoolers. The physician should also ask to whom the psychologist would recommend referral, if psychiatric backup should be needed.

One final note: if a child is suspected of multiple handicaps, the physician may wish to refer to a large medical center for a comprehensive interdisciplinary evaluation.

INFORMATION TO SUPPLY ON REFERRAL

Since the psychologist is able to evaluate only a small sample of the child's behavior, information provided by the physician is very important. On referral the physician should provide the following:

1. all relevant information regarding the child's impairments;
2. significant elements in the prenatal and postnatal history;

3. any medications which could affect behavior; and
4. the precise concern—mental, physical, or emotional—for which the child is being referred.

An actual case history of a child who was referred for a psychological evaluation is presented as Appendix A of this chapter. It provides an example of the kind of information which the primary care physician should provide to the psychologist upon referral.

PARENTAL RESPONSE

One final point that should be remembered is that it may often be necessary for the physician to play an active role in getting the parents to follow through on referral to a psychologist. Parents may be concerned about their role in the child's problem or may be afraid of what is wrong with the child. Parents also frequently feel guilty about being a "bad" parent or may have significant grief about their child's handicaps so that it is difficult for them to follow through on a referral.

The physician will probably want to discuss with the psychologist how the results should be reported to the parents. Most psychologists will prefer to be involved in interpreting the findings to parents and in helping parents work through such emotional reactions as grief.

SUMMARY

In summary, this chapter has discussed a number of ways the psychologist can assist the primary care physician. The psychologist can help assess or identify a child's disability or emotional difficulty, can help evaluate how much of the problem stems from familial relationships, can help counsel parents, and can serve as an advocate for children needing services.

APPENDIX A

Case History

Angela is a 45-month-old girl who was brought for a developmental evaluation to a child development center by her parents, who wanted to know the nature and extent of her developmental problem.

At birth, Angela was a 1,940 gram, small-for-gestational-age term infant, born via cesarean-section (due to breech presentation and failure of progression of labor). Neonatal problems included early rupture of the membranes, and jaundice that required no specific therapy. Angela was discharged after nine hospital days, apparently in good health. The only other known problem during the pregnancy or neonatal course was a questionable maternal seizure during the fifth month of pregnancy.

Angela did well by history until 18 months of age, when she developed a grand mal type seizure disorder. A rather extensive investigation performed at that time revealed no specific etiology. Subsequently, the seizures were reasonably well controlled initially with phenobarbital, which was discontinued because of hyperactivity; presently the seizures are being controlled with dilantin and meboral. Angela is presently followed in the Birth Defects Clinic and the Neurology Clinic of Colorado General Hospital. She is currently receiving speech therapy.

In addition to the above facts, there is no family history of mental retardation. There has been a great deal of denial and resistance to evaluation of the patient on the part of the family. The parents feel the patient is "normal;" but this denial is gradually diminishing, and the family, at this time, seems more amenable to therapeutic intervention. The parents report concern about Angela's short attention span and their difficulty in knowing what she understands. They feel that she is in constant motion and needs an extreme amount of attention.

Physical examination did not indicate any gross visual or auditory deficits. Angela's gross motor skills are at approximately the 30-month level, reflecting an 18-month delay with some indication of central nervous system impairment or dysfunction. She also shows significantly delayed expressive and receptive language skills. Her behavior is difficult to manage and her attention span is very short. Three months ago Angela's parents placed her in a special preschool for help with these problems.

A psychological evaluation is requested to determine:

1. What is Angela's current level of intellectual functioning and what type of intervention would be most appropriate?
2. Are there significant emotional factors that have contributed to her developmental delay, and are they secondary to other causes?
3. How can the parents be helped to understand her problems and manage her behavior?
4. Is Angela hyperactive?

BIBLIOGRAPHY

Johnston, R., and Magrab, P. *Developmental disorders: Assessment, treatment, and education.* Baltimore: University Park Press, 1977.

Palmer, J. O. *The psychological assessment of children.* New York: John Wiley and Sons, 1970.

Schnell, R. Special learning problems of young children. In J. Travers (Ed.), *The new children.* Stamford, Conn.: Greylock, 1976.

Ulrey, G. Psychological testing of young children. In J. Travers (Ed.), *The new children.* Stamford, Conn.: Greylock, 1976.

Chapter 12

Goal

To develop skills in identification and treatment of children who have been abused and neglected.

Objectives

At the end of this chapter, the physician should be able to:

- discuss the high relationship between child abuse and neglect and developmental disabilities;
- state the signs and symptoms of both child abuse and neglect so as to correctly suspect the mistreatment of children;
- state the proper steps to take when child abuse and/or neglect are suspected.

ABUSE AND NEGLECT EVALUATION

By
HAROLD P. MARTIN, M.D.

I. Introduction
   A. More than half of all abused and neglected children demonstrate problems in development.
   B. A conservative estimate of the prevalence of child abuse and neglect in the United States is that one percent of children are abused during their lifetimes, and that the frequency of neglect is at least twice as high.
   C. Many of the developmental disabilities of mistreated children can be prevented through early identification and intervention.
II. Definition
   Child abuse is defined by the U.S. Congress as "the physical or mental injury, sexual abuse, negligent treatment or maltreatment of a child under the age of 18 by a person who is responsible for the child's welfare under circumstances which indicate that the child's health or welfare is harmed or threatened thereby."
III. Symptoms and Signs of Child Abuse
   A. Common findings which should make the physician suspect physical abuse include multiple injuries or fractures, especially when at different stages of healing.
   B. Injuries in child abuse cases are frequently not adequately explained by the history, the history may be vague or conflicting, or the parents may keep changing the history.
   C. There may be a history of repeated "accidents."
   D. The parents may have delayed in seeking medical aid for the child's injuries.
   E. There may be pathognomonic lesions or retinal hemorrhages.
   F. There may be unusual parental behavior, including anger at the child, inappropriate expectations, and so forth.
IV. Initial Work-Up and Management of Child Abuse
   A. In all 50 states the physician is required to report a suspicion of abuse or neglect to a state agency.
   B. The physician is not required to make a diagnosis of abuse; the legal decision of abuse is delegated to social agencies.
   C. The first step a physician must take when abuse is suspected is to report orally within 24 hours to the appropriate agency; an official form must be filled out and submitted within 48 hours.
   D. The physician must give immediate attention to injuries and wounds.
   E. Screening should be conducted for a potential bleeding disorder.
   F. A skeletal survey should be obtained for children under five years of age.
   G. A complete physical examination is required, and exact measurements and descriptions of the injuries must be made.
   H. The child must be provided with an immediate place of safety, either in a hospital or foster home; arrangements for such placement can be made by the physician or social agencies.

V. Long-Term Management of the Abused Child
  A. The developmental status of the abused child must be observed so that a diagnosis of possible delays can be obtained.
  B. The physician should examine the siblings of the abused child.
  C. Medical problems common to abused children must be sought, and if identified, treated.
  D. Psychological crisis intervention is indicated for the child.
  E. Within a week, the case should be discussed at an interdisciplinary child abuse team meeting.
  F. Long-term intervention can include therapeutic day care or a therapeutic preschool, specific therapies, and medical and developmental follow-up.
  G. Assistance for the parents can include homemaker services, a parents' group, marital counseling, education in child-rearing practices, and so forth.
VI. Symptoms and Signs of Child Neglect
  A. Because neglect is not as clearcut a syndrome as abuse, the physician should consider whether the child's condition is due to parental inattention, and whether the child is in a safe and healthy environment.
  B. The physician plays an important role in suspecting neglect, but the legal determination of neglect is made by a social agency.
  C. Since abuse and neglect are often both present, all the signs and symptoms listed for child abuse may be found in the neglected child.
  D. Physical findings in cases of child neglect include poor physical growth, neglected hygiene and physical care, insufficient medical attention for past and present illnesses, a history of inadequate diet, a history of inadequate stimulation, an apathetic or irritable child, or parents who do not demonstate the usual caring behaviors.
  E. Neglect does not always stem from a parent's rejection of a child; neglect can be caused by a mother ignorant of child-crafting skills, or overwhelmed by social, family, economic, and psychological stresses.
VII. Initial Work-Up and Management of Child Neglect
  A. The initial workup for a child suspected of being neglected is quite similar to that for the abused child; the physician should consider coincident abuse.
  B. A history of ingestions should be obtained.
  C. When the presenting concern is failure to thrive, the child should be hospitalized and fed an age-appropriate diet to see if there is a spurt in weight gain during the first 10 days; only routine laboratory work should be conducted on admission.
VIII. Long-Term Management of the Neglected Child
  A. The steps outlined under management of the abused child are also indicated for the neglected child.
  B. When the neglect is secondary to overwhelming social stress, there is a need for concrete help, such as homemaking services, job training, child care, and so forth.
  C. A young mother may need parent education and individual support; an emotionally overwhelmed mother may need psychiatric help and assistance with child care.
IX. Identifying Abuse and Neglect in the Delayed Child
  A. When a physician encounters a developmentally delayed child and wonders if the etiology is mistreatment, four diagnostic clues can be sought.
  B. The physician should look for a history of past accidents or traumas; usually the parents will reveal these, if asked.
  C. The physician should look for signs of current or past trauma on the physical examination.

    D. The quality of the parent-child relationship is the most important clue; parents may show that they do not have much interest in their child, that they do not like the child, that they have minimal interaction with the child, and/or that they have unduly high expectations of the child.

    E. In addition, parents may be oriented toward whether the child is compliant rather than happy; discipline is apt to be harsh and erratic.

    F. The personality traits of a mistreated child may be another diagnostic clue; the mistreated child is usually unhappy, and at one end of the behavioral spectrum or the other.

    G. The mistreated child usually relates to other people in unusual ways; even if the child is attached to the parents, the relationship still is apt to be somewhat deviant.

X. Prevention of Developmental Disabilities

    A. The basis for most of the developmental delays demonstrated by abused and neglected children is the pattern of parenting to which they have been exposed, rather than to injury or medical neglect.

    B. The younger the child at the time of intervention, the greater the chances of reversing developmental delays; a change of parenting patterns can be accomplished by alternate care or by intervening with the biological parents.

    C. At least 75 percent of mistreated children can safely remain with their biological parents, or can be returned to them in less than six months.

    D. When foster care is required, the child should have frequent contact with the parents; the exception to this is when an early decision is made to remove the child from the parents.

XI. Impedances to Identification and Treatment

    A. If unchecked, strong emotional responses of physicians can interfere with proper care of an abused or neglected child.

    B. Anger is a common response; the physician who feels anger building toward mistreating parents should ask another professional to help deal with them.

    C. Many physicians erroneously believe that well-educated, middle class parents are not capable of mistreatment; child abuse and neglect knows no social boundaries.

    D. Some physicians are cynical regarding reporting suspected abuse or neglect to a social agency; it should be remembered that these agencies in most instances do a better job than any other agency or professional can.

XII. Summary

INTRODUCTION

A lesson on child abuse and neglect is included in this text because of the high relationship between mistreated children and developmental disabilities. More than 50 percent of abused and neglected children demonstrate problems in development, including: impaired intelligence; learning disabilities; specific developmental delays, especially in language and gross motor development; and psychological problems, many of which contribute to the delays and impairments in development noted above.

Child abuse and neglect are not uncommon in the United States. A conservative estimate would be that one percent of children in the U.S. are abused during their lifetimes, and the frequency of child neglect is at least twice as high. Hence, mistreatment of children is a significant etiology of developmental disabilities. In a recent study of 140 admissions to a residential facility for retarded children, it was found that three percent of the children were definitively retarded due to physical abuse. At least 11 percent of the children *might* have been retarded due to physical abuse, and 22 percent had independent professional evidence of prior abuse—whether it was etiological or not. Forty-eight percent of the retarded youngsters had been neglected. In 24 percent of the 140 children, neglect was felt to be a contributory factor in reduced intellectual potential.

A second rationale relates to the preventive aspects of identifying abuse and neglect. Many of the developmental disabilities of mistreated children can be prevented through early identification and intervention by the physician.

DEFINITION

Child abuse is defined by the U.S. Congress as "the physical or mental injury, sexual abuse, negligent treatment or maltreatment of a child under the age of 18 by a person who is responsible for the child's welfare under circumstances which indicate that the child's health or welfare is harmed or threatened thereby."

SYMPTOMS AND SIGNS OF CHILD ABUSE

The following are common findings which should make the physician suspect physical abuse:

1. There are multiple injuries or fractures, especially when at different stages of healing.
2. The injury(s) is not adequately explained by the history.
3. The history is vague or the parents tell conflicting stories or keep changing the history.
4. There is a history of repeated "accidents."
5. The parents have delayed in seeking medical care for the child's injuries.
6. There are such pathognomonic lesions as cigarette burns, cord or belt-buckle

marks, bites, strap marks, grab marks, or trauma in the front of the mouth due to forced feeding.
7. There are retinal hemorrhages. (When there are no skull fractures or signs of trauma about the head, these are usually due to severe shaking of the child.)
8. There is unusual parental behavior. These include parents who: disappear during hospital admission; show anger at the child for the injuries; do not visit the child in the hospital; show signs of rejecting the child; have highly inappropriate expectations for the child considering his or her age.

INITIAL WORK-UP AND MANAGEMENT OF CHILD ABUSE

In all 50 states, the physician is required to report a *suspicion* of abuse or neglect to a state agency—usually the Child Protection Services (CPS) or the local police department. It is important to note that the physician is neither requested nor required to make a *diagnosis* of abuse; rather, the physician is required to report a family when the possibility of mistreatment seems likely or highly probable. The physician may be able to state that a child's injuries are due to inflicted trauma; whether or not that injury constitutes child abuse is a community decision (made by the courts, by the assigned community agencies, such as CPS, or by the police). The physician's findings and impressions are critically important in making a decision of child abuse, but neither child abuse nor neglect are medical diagnoses. Instead, they are diagnoses which society makes through its elected or appointed representatives.

Given this background, the following steps should be taken when the physician suspects physical abuse.

First, the physician needs to report (orally within 24 hours, and in writing within 48 hours) to the appropriate community agency. There is an official form in each state which is to be filled out by the physician.

Second, the immediate injuries and wounds need attention.

Third, screening for a potential bleeding disorder is indicated. If the case comes to court later, the parents may contend that the bruises could be due to easy bruising or to an undiagnosed bleeding diathesis.

Fourth, a skeletal survey should be obtained in children under five years of age, or in any child who cannot tell the physician of tenderness or past injuries. The metaphysis, or subperiosteal bleeding, are tip-offs to inflicted injury. (X-rays taken two weeks after the injury may show callus formation or metaphyseal fragmentation when the original X-ray was only questionable.)

Fifth, complete physical examination—not just an examination of the obvious injury—is essential. The physician should look for hidden injuries, such as inside the mouth, under the hair, or in the retina. The genitals and anal region must be examined.

Sixth, exact measurements and descriptions of the injuries are essential. Photographs of the injuries will often be helpful if testimony in court is required at a later date.

And seventh, the child must be provided with an immediate place of safety. If the physician cannot be sure that it is safe to allow the child to return home, alternate care must be arranged. Hospitalization is often utilized for safety as well as for the advantage of giving the physician and CPS workers two to three days of time in which to investigate the family and home. Such an investigation is often necessary to determine whether or not the child has been mistreated. If the family does not agree to hospitalization, a 48-hour court hold should be obtained immediately. If the physician does not want to call the local judge, hospital social services can arrange this; or the community's CPS worker can be asked to obtain a 48-hour court hold for the child. An alternative to hospitalization is emergency foster home care, which can be arranged by the local CPS worker.

LONG-TERM MANAGEMENT OF THE ABUSED CHILD

The abused child must be observed and his or her developmental status and personality screened. This may be done by hospital staff members if the child is hospitalized. If the child is not in a hospital, this may be arranged by the primary care physician or by the responsible CPS worker. As noted in other chapters, if screening for development or personality is suspect or abnormal, then psychological consultation and comprehensive evaluations will be required for exact diagnosis.

The siblings of the abused child should be seen and examined by a physician. While only one child in a particular family may be mistreated, it is more common for several or all children in a family to be the victims of mistreatment.

The abused child is at increased risk for a number of medical problems in addition to the acute injuries. Those problems should be identified and treated. Especially common are anemia, infections, poor nutrition, hearing loss (often mild to moderate), inadequate immunizations, and other signs of past medical neglect.

Psychological crisis intervention is indicated for the child. Someone should be assigned the task of talking to the child during the days and weeks after a diagnosis of abuse; such crisis intervention is similar to that suggested for the child who has lost a parent. The counselor should listen to the child, and clarify the distorted ideas the child has as to why he or she was injured and removed from the parents. The counselor—who may be the physician or a CPS worker—must remember that the child has to deal with the pain of injuries, placement in a hospital or foster care setting, separation from the parents, possibly an appearance in court, and so forth.

Within a week, the case should be discussed at an interdisciplinary child abuse team meeting. At this time information from all concerned—the physician as well as a CPS worker and other consultants—can be pooled to plan for long-term treatment for the child and the family.

Long-term intervention for the child often includes the following approaches.

1. Therapeutic day care or a therapeutic preschool, which can attend to the child's developmental delays and psychological problems, may be ar-

ranged. This approach may also make it possible for the child to remain with the parents, for some parents may be able to adequately care for the child if care is not required 24 hours per day.

2. The child may require one or more specific therapies, such as speech therapy, special education, physical therapy, individual psychotherapy, etc.

3. Medical and developmental follow-up for the child should be arranged at the planning conference by the interdisciplinary team.

The child and his or her siblings are not the only family members in need of assistance; a combination of services will be needed by the parents. Exact treatment needs to be specifically planned, but should include some combination of the following:

1. casework;
2. homemaker services;
3. a lay-therapist for the primary caregiver;
4. a parents' group, such as Parents Anonymous;
5. assistance with child care;
6. marital counseling;
7. help with job placement, housing, money management, and so forth;
8. parent education in child rearing practices;
9. psychotherapy for either parent;
10. some form of assistance which focuses on nurturance and understanding for the parent(s).

SYMPTOMS AND SIGNS OF CHILD NEGLECT

Neglect is not as clearcut a syndrome as abuse. The signs and symptoms are less sharply defined, and the legal definition is less clear. The guiding rule of thumb is for the physician to first consider whether the child's condition may be due to parental inattention, and to next consider whether the child is in a safe and healthy environment.

As with abuse, the decision as to whether a child's condition constitutes neglect is an issue for society to decide.

The physician plays an important role in suspecting neglect, and in determining whether the child's condition is due to parental inattention. An example of this might be a child found to be suffering from heatstroke after being left unattended in a closed automobile. The physician may justifiably feel that the child should not have been left alone in this situation. However, the community must decide whether or not this legally constitutes child neglect.

Abuse and neglect are often both present. At least 10 percent of neglected children are also physically abused; conversely, approximately one-third of all abused children have signs of child neglect. Hence, *any* of the signs and symptoms listed for child abuse may be found in the neglected child.

There are various forms of neglect, including emotional neglect. The most pertinent issue for the primary care physician is the identification of "physical" neglect, e.g., neglect of medical care, nutrition, hygiene, and so on.

One common finding is of poor physical growth based on inadequate calorie or protein intake. Failure to thrive is the most common syndrome. Weight is more affected than height, falling more quickly when calories are inadequate; weight and/or height may be more than two standard deviations below the mean. However, equal concern is raised when the *rate* of weight gain is diminishing, even if the actual measurement does not plot out more than two standard deviations below the mean.

The neglected child usually has numerous signs of neglect of hygiene and physical care. These may include diaper rash, a dirty and unkempt appearance, malodor, garments smelling of urine or feces, and so forth.

Another common finding involves failure to provide medical attention for past or current illnesses.

There may be a history of inadequate diet. The physician may find, through questioning, that convenience foods are a mainstay of the child's diet.

In addition, there may be a history of inadequate stimulation. The parent may not talk to the child, play with the child, or provide play opportunities or toys for the child.

The neglected child is usually apathetic or irritable, giving evidence of not having learned to enjoy interaction with others. In addition, many neglectful parents do not demonstrate the usual caring behaviors. They may not touch or comfort the child, may not look at the child, may not talk with the child, and so forth.

This last point raises an important issue. Neglect does not always stem from a parent's rejection of a child, although that is a common phenomenon. Indeed, the parent may not seem to like the child, and may give evidence of rejection. However, neglect may also occur for other reasons which do not stem from an inherent lack of investment in the child.

The child's basic needs may be neglected out of ignorance of child-crafting skills, especially when a young mother with her first child is involved.

Another type of neglect occurs in families where the mother (as the primary caregiver) is overwhelmed by social, family, and economic stresses, and has little energy, time, or resources to use in caring for the child. This kind of mother may have the capacity for love and caring, but a low income, a large family, marital instability, or other stresses may sap her time and energy.

A fourth type of neglect occurs when a mother is overwhelmed with psychological stress; such a mother is just not available to the child. This is most often seen when the mother is depressed, and thus cannot attend to another person, including her dependent infant.

The physician's concern regarding neglect does not stem from a judgmental criticism of a parent—for the parent may not be able to adequately care for the child for reasons which are quite understandable. One need not see any evidence of a malevolent parenting style to suspect neglect. Rather, the physician must take the position of concern for whether the child is adequately cared for—regardless of the reason—and hence whether intervention needs to occur. One's concern must be whether or not the child is in a safe and healthy environment, not whether the parents are loving or rejecting the child.

INITIAL WORK-UP AND MANAGEMENT OF CHILD NEGLECT

The initial work-up for a child suspected of being neglected is quite similar to that for the abused child. A few differences need emphasis. These are as follows.

1. When neglect is suspected, the physician should also consider coincident abuse. Hence, a complete physical examination and a radiologic bone survey should be done in the child under five years of age.
2. A history of ingestions should be obtained, since ingestions are often secondary to parental neglect.
3. When the presenting concern is undernutrition, growth failure, or failure to thrive, the child should be hospitalized. Only routine laboratory work should be conducted on admission, and the child should be fed a routine, age-appropriate diet. A spurt in weight gain starting within the first 10 days is diagnostic. Occasionally neglected children have learned to not eat; in such cases, the physician may need a psychological consultation to help the child unlearn the aversion to feeding.

LONG-TERM MANAGEMENT

The eight steps outlined under management of the abused child are also indicated for the neglected child.

In the neglect syndrome, there is a more obvious need for concrete help for the family in homemaking services, job training, child care, and so forth—especially when the neglect is secondary to overwhelming social stress. Parental education and individual support may be what is needed in the young mother who has not learned child-crafting skills. Psychiatric help may be needed for the emotionally overwhelmed mother, in addition to assistance with child care until the mother's mental health has been returned.

IDENTIFYING ABUSE AND NEGLECT IN THE DELAYED CHILD

Most of this chapter has discussed the physician suspecting, diagnosing, and caring for a child at or near the time when mistreatment has taken place. This has been emphasized because of the critical importance of recognizing abuse and neglect, and of preventing developmental disabilities which are likely to occur if mistreatment goes unrecognized. However, there is another aspect to the identification of abuse and neglect; this involves the dilemma the physician faces when he or she recognizes that a child is developmentally disabled, and wonders if past abuse or neglect might be the cause.

The physician in this latter situation should look for four diagnostic clues. The first is to look for a history of past accidents or traumas. The parents will not be likely to admit that they have abused their child in the past, but will probably reveal their child's past fractures, injuries, or falls.

A second clue to look for is signs of trauma on the physical examination. These traumas may be current, or may be from the past.

The third and most important diagnostic clue is the quality of the parent-child relationship. Abuse and neglect result from a deviant parent-child relationship. Therefore, unless there has been successful intervention which has changed the parents' feelings and behaviors towards their child, some of the following would be expected to be noted.

1. Parents may show, verbally or through their actions, that they do not have much interest or investment in the child.
2. Parents may be interested in their child, but may make it clear that they do not like the child, or that they disapprove of the child.
3. Parents may not be able to think of things about the child which they enjoy.

4. Parents will usually show minimal affectionate behavior for the child, and will usually talk very little with the child.
5. Parents may have unduly high expectations of their child.
6. Parents may be primarily oriented toward whether the child is good or compliant, rather than focusing on what the child enjoys and whether the child is happy.
7. Parents probably employ harsh and uncompromising discipline. The discipline may also be quite erratic, so that a particular behavior of the child is met on occasion with approval, at other times with no response, and at still other times with verbal or physical attack.

The fourth diagnostic clue a physician should employ is to recognize personality traits of the child which *might* suggest deviant parenting. While there is no pathognomonic personality of an abused or neglected child, there are several traits which recur time and time again in mistreated children.

1. The mistreated child is nearly always an unhappy child. It is very rare to see an abused or neglected child who is happy, who enjoys age-appropriate play, or who has a good concept of him- or herself.
2. The mistreated child is usually at one end of the spectrum or the other on behavioral profiles. For example, the child is apt to be either very neat and meticulous, or quite chaotic and disorganized; he or she may be either unusually complaint and cooperative, or may be quite oppositional and uncooperative.
3. The abused or neglected child generally has unusual qualities in relationships to other people. Probably most common is the child who is indiscriminately friendly to strangers, showing no evidence of the normal wariness or caution that should be seen. Slightly less often, one sees the abused child who is unduly fearful of strangers; this kind of child is a quiet, shy, frightened creature.

4. While the mistreated child may be attached to his or her parent(s), the relationship still is apt to be somewhat deviant. Again, the extremes of behavior should be looked for. The child may be unusually obedient and "disciplined"—or may be quite provocative and uncontrollable.

In summary, when seeing a child with developmental disabilities, it may be quite difficult to be sure whether the etiology could be abuse or neglect from months or years ago. A history given by the parents and perusal of old medical records may clarify that the child has had many injuries, whether or not parent culpability was considered when these occurred. The examination, in addition to possible signs of brain damage, may show signs of current or past trauma. The parent-child relationship may still be deviant, even if overt physical abuse or neglect are no longer operant, and the child's personality may reveal some signs of previous deviant parenting.

PREVENTION OF DEVELOPMENTAL DISABILITIES

More than 50 percent of abused and neglected children show evidence of developmental disabilities at the time of diagnosis. The earlier these disabilities—and the syndrome of maltreatment—are identified, the better is the prognosis for normal developmental function. The basis for most of these developmental delays is the pattern of parenting to which the abused or neglected child has been exposed—rather than being due to brain damage from injury or medical neglect. The younger the child when intervention begins, the greater the chances of reversing a developmental delay. A change in parenting can be accomplished by alternate care (such as foster placement) or by changing the care the biologic parents give to the child.

At least 75 percent of mistreated children can safely remain with their biologic parents, or can return to them after a relatively short (less than six months) stay in foster care. When foster care is needed, it is important that the child have frequent contact with the biological parents to minimize weakening the attachment between child and parents. The only exception to this is when an early decision is made that permanent relinquishment of parental rights is indicated. The continuation of the bond between parent and child should not be based on any "reward" to the parent for compliance in treatment recommendations, but is based on the needs of the child.

IMPEDANCES TO IDENTIFICATION AND TREATMENT

Child abuse and neglect engender a great deal of emotional reaction in everyone involved—including physicians. It is critically important that the primary care physician be aware of such feelings, inasmuch as they can, if unchecked, interfere with proper care of the child and family.

One common response is anger. The physician is likely to become quite angry at parents who have mistreated a child. The more severe or bizarre the injuries, the greater the potential for anger. It would probably be meaningless to try to convince a practitioner that he or she should not be angry at the parents, who were probably themselves mistreated as children. However, two points deserve emphasis. First, the majority of abusive parents do not want to mistreat their children. They want help to stop their mistreatment. The second point is that if the physician shows his or her anger towards the parents, it will make meaningful treatment for the child more difficult. When the physician sees an abused or neglected child and is aware that feelings of anger are building, someone else should be asked to help; a social worker or nurse, for example, can be asked to assist by interviewing the parents. It is not necessary, and often not possible, for any physician to be able to calmly and cooly handle an abuse or neglect case all alone.

Disbelief is another common reaction to child abuse and neglect. Many physicians just cannot believe that well-meaning people could seriously harm or neglect a child. This is especially true if the parents are similar to the physician—that is, if they are middle class, well-educated, and "nice" people. It is true that all adults are capable of mistreating a child; even people who care about their children are capable of mistreatment. This is very important to remember, as it relates to the reason that so few private physicians "see" or suspect child abuse in their middle class, private practices. For example, a few years ago in New York City, of more than 2,000 cases of abuse and neglect which were reported in one year, only seven were reported from practicing physicians. Middle class and upper class families can and do abuse and neglect their children, and they deserve help in their parenting as much as do low income families.

A third response among physicians when they confront the possibility of abuse or neglect is cynicism. Physicians may feel that the identification of abuse and neglect will not lead to any good things happening for the child and family. This may explain why some physicians will not report suspect cases to social agencies, but instead try to handle such cases themselves (perhaps with the assistance of a mental health referral). Admittedly, social service agencies do not always handle cases of abuse and neglect as well as one might wish. Nonetheless, considering the hundreds of cases most counties handle a year, they do a much better job than any other agency or professional can. They should and usually do take a "helping" stance towards the family—not a punitive or accusatory position. They try to arrange whatever assistance is needed to help a family stop abusive or neglectful behavior, and to provide an adequate home for the child. In most instances, they are successful.

SUMMARY

The history of recognition of child maltreatment stemmed from Dr. C. Henry Kempe's landmark papers in 1961 when the term "battered child" was coined. The number of children who have been recognized as maltreated has mushroomed since then. For example, in Colorado during 1970, only 120 cases of suspected abuse or neglect were reported. Seven years later, almost 4,000 cases were reported in Colorado. This pattern has been mimicked in every state.

The last few years of the 1970s has emphasized the morbidity of abuse and neglect. Developmental disabilities and emotional distress in the victims is now being recognized. The generational transmission of abuse and neglect are now known, and highlight the importance of diagnosis and treatment as a preventive measure against future generations of children being mistreated.

The child's physician plays an important role in recognizing suspected cases of child abuse and neglect. He or she is the professional who will most likely appreciate the symptoms and signs of these syndromes. In addition, the physician plays a critically important advocacy role in raising questions as to the child's developmental status, and in making recommendations to the CPS agency and/or the court as to what intervention is necessary for remediation of developmental delays.

In the majority of instances, the child's family can be kept intact. The child's developmental status will only be assured if the physician emphasizes the need for treatment to be directed at changing the parenting style in the family—and if the physician insists on treatment for the mistreated child's developmental problems.

BIBLIOGRAPHY

Buchanan, A., and Oliver, J. F. Abuse and neglect as a cause of mental retardation. *British Journal of Psychiatry,* 1977, *131,* 458–467.

Elmer, E., and Gregg, G. S. Developmental characteristics of abused children. *Pediatrics,* 1967, *40,* 596–602.

Goldson, E., Fitch, M. J., Wendell, T. A., and Knapp, G. Child abuse: Its relationship to birthweight, Apgar score, and developmental testing. *American Journal of Diseases in Children,* 1978, *132,* 790–793.

Gregg, G. S., and Elmer, E. Infant injuries: Accident or abuse. *Pediatrics,* 1969, *44,* 434–439.

Helfer, R., and Kempe, C. H. (Eds.). *The battered*

child (3rd ed.). Chicago: University of Chicago Press, 1981.

Hufton, I. W., and Oates, R. K. Non-organic failure to thrive: A long-term follow-up. *Pediatrics, 1977, 59,* 73–77.

Hunter, R. S., Kilstrom, N., Kraybill, E. N., and Loda, F. Antecedents of child abuse and neglect in premature infants: A prospective study in a newborn intensive care unit. *Pediatrics, 1978, 61,* 629–635.

Kempe, C. H. Approaches to preventing child abuse: The health visitors concept. *American Journal of Diseases in Children, 1976, 130,* 941–947.

Kerns, D. L. Child Abuse and Neglect. The pediatrician's role. *Journal of Continuing Education, Pediatrics,* 1979, 21(7), 11–27.

Lewis, D. O., Shanok, S. S., Pincus, J. H., and Glaser, G. H. Violent juvenile delinquents: Psychiatric, neurological, psychological, and abuse factors. *Journal of American Academy of Child Psychiatry,* 1979, *18,* 307–319.

McKay, H., Sinisterra, L., McKay, A., Gomez, H., and Lloreda, P. Improving cognitive ability in chronically deprived children. *Science,* 1978, *200,* 270–278.

Martin, H. P. The child and his development. In C. H. Kempe and R. Helfer (Eds.), *Helping the battered child and his family,* Philadelphia: J. B. Lippincott Company, 1972.

Martin, H. P. (Ed.) *The abused child: An interdisciplinary approach to developmental issues and treatment.* Cambridge, Mass.: Ballinger, 1976.

Martin, H. P. The abuse and neglect of children. *Comprehensive Therapy,* 1979, *5,* 57–61.

Martin, H. P. *User manual on upgrading child abuse and neglect programs: treatment of abused and neglected children.* Washington, D.C.: National Center on Child Abuse and Neglect, ACYF, HEW, 1979.

Martin, H. P., and Beezley, P. Behavioral observations of abused children. *Developmental Medicine/Child Neurology,* 1977, *19,* 373–387.

Martin, H. P., Beezley, P., Conway, E. F., and Kempe, C. H. The development of abused children. *Advances in Pediatrics,* 1974, *21,* 25–73.

Ryan, M. G., Davis, A. A., and Oates, R. K. 187 cases of child abuse and neglect. *Medical Journal of Australia,* 1977, *2,* 623–628.

Sandgrund, A., Gaines, R. W., and Green, A. H. Child abuse and mental retardation: A problem of cause and effect. Journal of Mental Deficiency, 1975, *19,* 327–330.

Schmitt, B. D. Battered child syndrome. In C. H. Kempe, H. K. Silver, and D. O'Brien (Eds.), *Current pediatric diagnosis and treatment* (5th ed.). Los Altos: Lange, 1978.

Smith, S. M., and Hanson, R. 134 battered children: A medical and psychological study. *British Medical Journal,* 1974, 666–670.

Chapter 13

Goal
To develop an awareness of the alternatives available to collate information from referral sources.

Objectives
At the end of this chapter, the physician should be able to:
- explain the importance of integrating diagnostic evaluations and recommendations for treatment;
- discuss various methods of assembling consultants according to the complexity of a case.

INTEGRATION OF DIAGNOSTIC FINDINGS

By
STEVEN POOLE, M.D.

I. Introduction
The case review serves the important function of compiling and integrating: diagnostic information from more than one discipline; treatment recommendations; methods of monitoring the child's progress.

II. The Physician's Role
A. The physician may opt to function as case manager or consultant.
B. Besides having responsibility for assessing physical needs, the physician can assist in the areas of family functioning and psychosocial problems.

III. The Case Manager's Role
A. The case manager compiles assessments and coordinates recommendations for treatment.
B. The case manager also oversees the parent conference, monitors implementation of treatment, and reevaluates the child's progress at a specified interval.

IV. Methods of Assembling Data
A. In a simple case (where up to three professionals are involved, findings are relatively straightforward, and there are no complex psychosocial problems), data can be gathered by mail or telephone.
B. In a complex case (where many professionals are involved, there are conflicting assessments and multiple delays, or where there are multiple family problems), it is usually necessary for an interdisciplinary conference to be held.

V. Conducting an Interdisciplinary Conference
A. An interdisciplinary case conference brings together all the specialists and takes between 60 and 90 minutes.
B. If not all the specialists are available, those who are most heavily involved should be included.

VI. Summary

INTRODUCTION

Whether a child has been seen by the physician and only one other specialist, or by the physician and several specialists, it is extremely important for all findings and recommendations to be collected and integrated. Too often when a child is referred to various specialists for evaluations there is no subsequent combination of findings and recommendations into a coherent plan. This integration process generally requires a case manager. The primary care physician is often the ideal person to gather the diagnostic information and, with the assistance of the evaluating consultants, to develop a realistic plan for management and treatment of the handicapped child.

THE PHYSICIAN'S ROLE

The primary care physician may decide to function as case manager or may choose the role of consultant. For the physician who is functioning as a consultant, there are several areas of responsibility within the traditional medical domain: the medical history; the physical examination (including vision, hearing, and a traditional neurological screening); assessment of genetic diseases; assessment of metabolic diseases; utilization of appropriate medical consultants; and integration of assessments and recommendations. In addition, the physician may also have much to contribute in the area of family functioning and psychosocial problems, since a continued relationship with the child's family provides the opportunity to learn much about these important matters.

THE CASE MANAGER'S ROLE

For the person who functions as case manager, there are a number of other responsibilities:

1. coordinating various specialists' evaluations;
2. integrating the evaluations and recommendations into a coherent plan;
3. overseeing the parent conference;
4. ensuring that someone is available to the family for communication regarding treatment, the monitoring process, reevaluation, and problem solving;
5. overseeing and monitoring the implementation of the plan and assigning responsibilities to the various specialists involved in treatment;
6. arranging for and following through with reevaluation at a specific interval;
7. solving problems during the treatment period.

METHODS OF ASSEMBLING DATA

In assembling and coordinating evaluations and recommendations, there are two basic approaches which a physician can take. The physician can:

1. accumulate data without actually meeting with the various specialists (utilizing written reports or telephone communication);
2. arrange for an interdisciplinary conference at which all professionals can discuss data and recommendations, and together develop a coherent treatment plan.

Because no one approach is best for all cases nor for all individuals, the approach to the collection and coordination of data should be selected with regard to the complexity of the case.

A simple case is one in which:

1. only one to three professionals are involved;
2. the findings are relatively straightforward;
3. there appears to be fairly close initial agreement between the various professionals regarding assessment and planning; or
4. there are no complex psychosocial problems, nor are there multiple problems within the family.

The complex case is the one in which:

1. there are more than three professionals involved;
2. the professionals hold conflicting opinions;
3. the child has multiple problems;
4. there are multiple problems within the family; or
5. there are limited resources available to the family.

Simple cases often lend themselves to case coordination via the telephone. For the complex case, an interdisciplinary conference is usually necessary. When initially confronted with what will probably evolve into a complex case, the physician may decide: to refer the child to an interdisciplinary developmental evaluation center; to identify someone else as the case manager; or to be case manager and assume responsibility for case coordination and the case conference.

CONDUCTING AN INTERDISCIPLINARY CONFERENCE

The interdisciplinary case conference brings together all of the specialists to assemble data, discuss opinions, and develop a treatment plan. This conference, which usually takes 60 to 90 minutes, should be held after all evaluations are completed, but prior to the parent conference. The physician should schedule the interdisciplinary case conference outside of office hours so as not to be interrupted. If it is not possible for all the specialists to meet, the case manager should try to get those who have been most heavily involved in assessments or who will be involved in the treatment process to attend.

The author had a private pediatric practice in which approximately one significant developmental problem was identified a month, as well as a referral practice which generated approximately one evaluation per week. Most of the cases (approximately 65 to 75 percent) were simple rather than complex. For those children older than five year of age, the school was case manager. For children under five years of age whose cases were simple, the author usually was case manager. For complex cases involving children less than five years of age, the author usually began as case manager; however, at the interdisciplinary conference another person (someone more directly involved in treatment and therefore in close contact with the child during the treatment period) was chosen to be the on-going case manager.

For simple cases, the combination of written reports and telephone contacts best facilitated integration of data from other professionals. After collecting the written reports, the author called the individual professionals to discuss with them the various proposed treatment plans. The telephone call allowed for exchanging opinions and negotiating an optimal treatment plan.

For complex cases, the author utilized interdisciplinary conferences, which were scheduled before office hours, at lunch, or after office hours on a quiet evening. The author found that meeting for a breakfast or lunch served as an enticement for getting the specialists together. Most families agreed that the physician ought to charge for this conference time.

The usual format of the interdisciplinary conference included:

1. an initial opportunity for each professional to present an evaluation and recommendations;
2. time for discussing the various recommendations;
3. an attempt to agree on a coherent plan; and
4. the assignment of responsibilities for various aspects of treatment—for a parent conference, for the monitoring of progress, and for the reevaluation.

SUMMARY

In summary, it is important for the primary care physician to consider the best way of coordinating each case in order to maximize the child's holistic health care. Two factors which should be kept in mind are: who will serve as the case manager; and how complex is the case. These factors will help the physician determine the approach that will best benefit the physician and the child.

Chapter 14

Goal   To increase the knowledge and skill level of the physician in conducting parent conferences.

Objectives   At the end of this chapter, the physician should be able to:
- identify the six goals of the initial parent conference;
- apply the six goals to clinical practice;
- describe how to terminate parent conference sessions.

PARENT CONFERENCES

By
HAROLD P. MARTIN, M.D.

I. Introduction
  The six goals of the initial parent conference are:
  1. Informing the parents of the diagnosis and etiology;
  2. Eliciting parents' cognitive and emotional responses;
  3. Responding to parents' questions and concerns;
  4. Assessing the effect on the family;
  5. Clarifying the physician's future role;
  6. Imparting a realistic perspective.
II. Informing the Parents
  A. During the initial parent conference, the physician informs the parents of the child's diagnosis, etiology, prognosis, and treatment.
  B. The parents will likely have an indication of the physician's concerns prior to the conference; nevertheless, the diagnosis can be expected to be a shock.
  C. The physician should tell the parents as much as possible about what did and did not cause the child's handicap.
III. Eliciting Parental Responses
  The physician must listen for and elicit both the parents' cognitive and emotional responses.
IV. Responding to the Parents
  Parents' questions and concerns must be responded to by the physician, even though the questions may not have been on the physician's agenda.
V. Assessing Effect on the Family
  The physician should note how the parents are responding to get some idea about how the family is apt to be affected by the handicapped child.
VI. Clarifying the Physician's Future Role
  A. Parents have been used to seeing the physician only for well child care or treatment during illnesses, and may not be sure what help the physician can give in the long term.
  B. Later questions which the parents may pose for the physician include questions about social relationships and the child's sexuality.
VII. Imparting a Realistic Perspective
  A. The physician should seek to give parents a realistic perspective of their child's condition and future.
  B. The physician should emphasize treatment which can help the child.
VIII. Conducting a Conference
  A. Individual styles which physicians have found to be successful in past dealings with families will probably work during parent conferences.
  B. The physician should frequently check the parents' emotional responses and understanding.

    C. The physician should be as personal as possible during a parent conference.

IX. Physicians' Affective Responses

    A. Physicians often feel sad, discouraged, and upset when confronted with a handicapped child; this is a natural reaction, for acknowledging that a child has a chronic problem may leave a physician feeling impotent.

    B. Physicians who do not recognize their own emotional responses to a disabled child may act inappropriately without realizing the reason for such behavior.

    C. It is important that physicians talk about their feelings with colleagues, spouses, or friends so that these emotional responses do not interfere with the practice of good medicine.

X. Parental Reactions

    A. Parents react to learning about their child's handicap much as they react to any life crisis.

    B. Parents may be overwhelmed and disoriented, they may not hear things clearly or express themselves clearly, and they may do or say things which are out of character.

    C. It is very common for parents to have misunderstood the physician during a parent conference.

    D. Other common parental reactions include denial, sorrow (or even depression), anger, and guilt.

    E. Families, upon learning of their child's disability, may function less well, but some may function the same or even better.

    F. The physician should identify and acknowledge parents' emotions during a conference.

XI. Planning a Parent Conference

    A. The conference should be scheduled after evaluation, when sufficient data on the child have been gathered.

    B. The initial and second parent conferences generally take between 30 and 60 minutes each.

    C. Conferences should be held when there will be no interruptions and in a place which provides privacy.

XII. Staffing a Parent Conference

    A. The primary care physician almost always is required to conduct the parent conference.

    B. Other professionals who attend should have a rapport with the parents and should be able to deal with parents' emotions.

    C. If the physician is unable to deal with the parents' emotional responses, another professional should be included in the conference.

XIII. The Second Parent Conference

    A. The second conference should follow the first by about a week, and requires about 30 minutes.

    B. The physician should learn the parents' understanding of information presented at the initial parent conference.

XIV. Ongoing Conferences

    A. Ongoing conferences give parents a chance to discuss their child's progress and to raise questions which have evolved.

    B. The physician can use the conferences to learn how the parents and family are being affected by the handicapped child.

XV. Terminating Parent Conferences

    A. Conferences should be terminated when the physician has imparted all the necessary information.

    B. Conferences should not be ended while the parents are still shocked and upset.

XVI. Summary

INTRODUCTION

The first parent conference is the time that a physician meets with the parents of a developmentally delayed child to discuss what is wrong with their child and what can be done about the child's condition. There are six goals which should be met during the initial parent conference. The first and most important goal is giving the parents information about their child. The second is to hear and understand the parents' cognitive and emotional responses to the information they have just received. The third is to respond to the parents' questions and concerns. Fourth is to try to anticipate how the family is apt to be affected by their developmentally delayed child. Fifth is to clarify the physician's future role with the family. And the last goal is to help the parents get a realistic perspective on both their child's developmental problems and strengths.

INFORMING THE PARENTS

The first stated goal, to inform the parents of their child's developmental problems, is the most important reason for meeting with the parents. The physician should inform them of at least four items. One is to inform them of the diagnosis; the parents must understand what is wrong with their child. Second is to discuss the etiology, the cause of the handicap. Third is to inform the parents about their child's prognosis. And fourth is to discuss the management or treatment of the problem.

The physician will most likely have given the family some indication of professional concerns prior to the first parent conference. Often the conference will be preceded by a number of consultations and examinations, perhaps including some laboratory tests. The parents will have become aware that the physician is concerned about the child's brain, intelligence, learning, motor ability, and so on. Therefore, the diagnosis should not come as a complete surprise to them. Nevertheless, at the first parent conference when the physician informs the parents of the diagnosis, there most likely will still be a reaction. The conference may be the first time that the concept of a particular handicap has really sunk in for the parents.

In discussing the etiology, the physician will not be able to make an exact diagnosis in at least half of the instances of developmental difficulties. However, the physician usually can either say something about the timing—whether the delay appears to be due to a problem during the pregnancy, at the time of labor and delivery, or after birth. This may be helpful. It may also be helpful for the physician to tell the parents what did *not* cause their child's problem. For example, the physician could tell them that such factors as chromosomal or biochemical abnormalities, genetic causes, or infections during pregnancy are not at fault.

Discussion at the initial parent conference should center on telling the parents what evaluations show is wrong with their child. It would be a mistake to spend a great deal of time discussing an exact prognosis over many years. However, the physician does need to tell the parents something about the significance of their child's disability. After all, parents do not necessarily know just what a diagnosis of cerebral palsy, aphasia, or mental retardation means. The physician needs to address the severity of the problem and how it is apt to affect the child now and for some time to come.

Finally, the physician needs to speak to the parents about management or treatment. What can be done to help the child? This is vitally important, because when parents learn that their child has a developmental problem or disability, they are likely to feel sad and hopeless. Because the physician is telling the parents that their child has an incurable lifelong problem, there is a real need for him or her to emphasize some positive aspects as well.

ELICITING PARENTAL RESPONSES

The second goal of the initial parent conference is to elicit and listen to the parents' responses. There are really two kinds of responses that the physician must listen for: the parents' cognitive responses and their emotional responses. The physician should check periodically during the conference to discover what the parents are hearing and understanding; it is very common for families to leave a parent conference having misunderstood and distorted much of the information given them. The physician also needs to check periodically to see how the parents are feeling.

RESPONDING TO THE PARENTS

The third goal of a parent conference is to respond to parents' queries. Clearly, the family will have a number of questions and concerns; some of these might touch on issues other than those the physician had planned. It is very important that the physician listen to those questions and concerns and respond to them—even though they may not have been on the original agenda.

ASSESSING EFFECT ON THE FAMILY

The fourth goal of a parent conference is for the physician to get some idea about how the family is apt to be affected. One of the best ways to evaluate this is by seeing how the parents are responding to the initial news about their child's developmental disability.

CLARIFYING THE PHYSICIAN'S FUTURE ROLE

A fifth goal of the parent conference is to clarify the physician's role in relation to the family. Most families have been used to seeing the physician only for well child care or for acute illnesses; they are not informed as to what help the physician can give them for their child's chronic, long-term developmental handicap.

For instance, as time goes on, the parents will have questions about their child's schooling. Other common questions include: what can parents do when their child is teased or called names by peers; or how should parents respond when the sibling of the child in question hesitates to bring friends home. Later, parents will have questions about the child's sexuality. The parents will not be sure whether these are questions the physician is willing to discuss with them, or whether—as has been the custom—they should continue to see the physician only for well child care and medical illnesses. Therefore, it is important that the physician clarify with the family what he or she will do over time.

IMPARTING A REALISTIC PERSPECTIVE

The final goal of a parental conference is to help the parents get a realistic perspective. Unfortunately, most of the information a physician delivers during the initial conference is bad news. The parents are told about a problem, an incurable condition; they need to know also that their child will continue to grow, develop, learn, and have friends. In short, the physician can emphasize the things which can be done to help the child.

CONDUCTING A CONFERENCE

The approach used by a physician in the initial parent conference is very important; as has been mentioned, much of this approach involves what has been said and done with the family long before the initial parent conference. During the evaluation, the physician has probably been asking questions which have given evidence of concerns to the family. Thus, before the initial parent conference the physician has laid some groundwork.

Part of the physician's approach in the parent conference has to do with individual styles. Each physician has his or her own style of talking to parents, of delivering information, and of counseling. Whatever style has been used successfully in past dealings with families will probably work during parent conferences.

The physician should approach the parent conference with two goals in mind: educating and counseling the parents, and helping them adjust to having a developmentally handicapped child. During these conferences, the physician must always try to be helpful to and supportive of the parents. One way the physician can do this is to stop periodically after giving the family some information. He or she can check back with the parents to see what they have heard, what they have understood, and what their emotional or affective responses are.

For instance, after telling the family about the diagnosis, the physician might stop and elicit parental responses. The physician could say something like: "I'm wondering what your reactions are to what I have just said?" or, "I wonder if this comes as a surprise to you? Is the diagnosis something you haven't expected?" The physician should do this "checking back" especially if he or she notices some affective response by either parent—some tears, facial sadness, staring into space, etc. With encouragement, the parents may tell the physician how they feel, may confess that the diagnosis doesn't make sense to them, or may ask questions.

It is also very important during the parent conference for the physician to be as personal as possible. Because, as has been noted, physicians usually have strong feelings and emotions about children with brain damage, retardation or chronic handicaps, there is often a tendency for physicians to depersonalize themselves. Each physician entering a parent conference must make a special effort to assure that depersonalization will not occur.

Little things can be very helpful to the parents. For example, the use of the child's name can be comforting. The physician should not say to the parents, "We've found that your child has a problem." Instead, he or she should say, "We've found that Sammy (or Sally) has a problem." The physician should remember that the purpose of the parent conference is not primarily to discuss the disease or condition; instead, it is to discuss with the parents the *child* who has a disease or condition.

PHYSICIANS' AFFECTIVE RESPONSES

Parents are not the only ones who may have strong feelings during a parent conference. It is especially important that physicians realize that they, themselves, also have feelings. If physicians who are talking and thinking about a child's problems often feel sad, discouraged, and upset, this is not hard to understand. It is not pleasant to acknowledge that a child has a chronic condition which will never go away; such a realization often leaves physicians feeling impotent. After all, most physicians have spent their lifetimes placing a high value on intelligence, on learning, and on competence—abilities handicapped children may never achieve.

The most important thing for physicians to recognize is their own emotional responses to a disabled child. When a physician does not recognize these reactions, he or she may act inappropriately, perhaps not realizing the reason for such behavior. This may be why some physicians bring up the possibility of institutionalizing a handicapped child even in the newborn period. It may also be the reason why physicians are sometimes curt and abrupt with the families of developmentally disabled children. The physician who is not in touch with his or her own feelings may schedule appointments for the child less frequently than would be optimal, in an unconscious attempt to avoid experiencing the feelings which are aroused by contact with the child and the family.

Many things in physicians' practices make them feel sad; for many physicians, seeing a child who is retarded or brain damaged is just such an instance. What is important is that physicians realize what they are feeling so that these emotional responses do not interfere with the practice of good medicine. Recognizing and talking with feelings about colleagues, spouses, or friends won't make the feelings go away—but may make them manageable and understandable.

PARENTAL REACTIONS

Parents react to learning that their child has a developmental handicap much as they react to any sort of life crisis. A general theory of crisis states that most families will go through some relatively predictable stages or reactions to stress or crisis; having a child who is retarded or brain damaged is in many respects no different from other kinds of major stresses. The intensity of the family's reaction will differ, and the length or duration of reactions will vary depending on the personality of the parents and the significance of the particular child's handicap.

Physicians should expect that the family will be overwhelmed during the parent conference, since most people, when confronted with crisis, become overwhelmed and often disoriented. They will not hear things clearly, they will not express themselves clearly, and they may do or say things they normally wouldn't. Although the parents may nod and act as if they understand the physician's comments, the news is often so overwhelming that it does not really register.

This is important for physicians to remember, since the family is later likely to ask questions that have been answered before. The parents may even claim that the physician has neglected to tell them something about their child—when they clearly *have* been told. The parents may need some repetition and clarification during several subsequent conferences.

Most people also react to crisis by manifesting some sort of denial. This may be very short-lived and relatively subtle, or it may be very pronounced. A few families, for instance, will "shop" from one physician to another, refusing to believe a painful diagnosis. These families find it difficult or even impossible to believe that their child has a disability. This state usually is relatively short-lived, but almost every parent of a handicapped child goes through it to some extent.

There are other very common reactions to stress that almost all people experience. Most parents, upon learning their child is handicapped, become sad; in some cases this sadness may turn into depression.

Anger is another reaction of almost all people to crisis. When parents suddenly realize that their child has a long-term, incurable problem, there is inevitably disappointment and some anger. That anger may be directed toward the child having a handicap, or it may be directed by the parents at themselves for having this problem. Usually parents are not very comfortable about being angry at the disabled child; after all, how can a parent blame Sammy or Sally for having Down Syndrome? So the anger is apt to be directed inappropriately and irrationally, sometimes toward the person who has delivered information about the handicap.

The parents may alternately display anger toward some other medical personnel, such as the obstetrician, or the nurses in the newborn nursery. Or parents may become angry with friends or relatives. In any case, the physician should be prepared for the parents to display irrational anger that they may not even identify in themselves.

Guilt is also usually felt to some degree by most families with developmentally delayed children. This is especially true when there is no diagnosis, because the parents are then very apt to feel that they might have caused the handicap, or that they might have been able to prevent it. What mother during pregnancy hasn't transgressed some of her obstetrician's rules? What expectant woman hasn't eaten some salty potato chips when she was on a low salt diet? What family hasn't had sexual intercourse after the obstetrician says to quit? Families may conjure up many irrational thoughts about their role in producing a handicapped child.

Most parents pass through the stages of sorrow, anger, and guilt fairly quickly. While there is often some remnant of these emotions for years, most families come to some healthy adaptation to the condition of their child. The physician must remember, however, that these initial reactions to the child's handicap may persist at a very low volume for a parent's lifetime. As a remnant of denial, there is often some unrealistic parental hope that the diagnosis was wrong, that some miracle cure will be found, or that the child will not really have the problems the physician predicts. At the very least, there will always be chronic sorrow for the parents of a disabled child, as they repeatedly face the reality that the handicapped child will never be able to do everything normal children can.

Physicians should recognize that after any crisis, families may function the same, less well, or better. The physician should not assume that the family will function less well simply because they have a child with a developmental handicap. Certainly, that is an option and a possibility; however, some parents adapt and actually improve their functioning as they become involved in the problem together.

How should physicians deal with families' emotional responses? Probably the most important concept for the physician to remember is the importance of identifying and acknowledging the parents' feelings. The physician will be able to see these emotions in both the initial parent conference and in subsequent conferences.

Therefore, the physician who sees a family acting in disbelief should acknowledge it; the physician might say something like, "I know this is hard to believe," or, "Perhaps you feel that I am wrong about your child's developmental problems?" When the physician sees signs of sadness, these should be acknowledged with such a phrase as, "I'm sure it's very difficult and makes you feel very sad to think about Sammy (or Sally) as slow in development." If the physician sees that the family is angry, this should also be acknowledged.

The physician should never pretend that a parent's emotion doesn't exist. Ignoring the family's sorrow, guilt, anger, and so on is likely to make the reaction longer and more intense. Usually the best thing a physician can do after acknowledging an emotion is simply to stop and let the family respond.

It is helpful for the family to be aware that their reactions and feelings are normal. They must be reassured that they

are not "crazy" or pathological because they are feeling extremely upset and overwhelmed, angry or sad. The problem is compounded if the mother and father believe they are the only parents who feel as they do, or that only "strange" people would react as they are reacting. Therefore, the physician should acknowledge both the emotional responses and the normalcy of them.

One principle physicians should follow is *not* to try to talk the parents out of their emotional reaction. It sometimes is tempting for the physician to say: "You really shouldn't be so sad about this. Sammy is just going to be a fine little boy, and he is going to be able to go to school and have a good life." While that may indeed be true, such a statement gives a message to the parents that they shouldn't experience sadness.

With anger, the temptation is to say, "Don't be so upset about what happened during the pregnancy, labor or delivery, or the way the neighbors are talking about your child." This kind of statement tells the family that there is something wrong with what they are feeling. It's a prohibition. The physician must acknowledge the normalcy of the parents' reaction, and should not try to take it away or prohibit it. It's apt to dissipate and to get less intense with time, for there is a natural course of adaptation to crisis. The physician will be most helpful to the parents in that normal course of adaptation by acknowledging, listening to, and responding to their reactions. (Appendix A contains items to serve as reminders during presentation of the videotaped parent conference demonstration.)

PLANNING A PARENT CONFERENCE

When is the best time for the initial parent conference? Obviously it must be after evaluation when sufficient data on the child have been gathered.

How long should the parent conference take? That varies, depending upon the style of the individual physician. On the average, however, the initial and follow-up parent conferences each will take between 30 and 60 minutes. The more serious and complex the problem, the more significant it will be to the family, and the longer a conference is likely to take.

Where should the parent conferences be held? It is very important that the first two parent conferences occur in a setting where there is appropriate dignity and solemnity to the problem being discussed. The parents should attend without the disabled child or siblings. The conference should be scheduled at a time when the physician will not be interrupted by visitors, patients, or phone calls. Some physicians set aside a certain portion of an afternoon in their practices for meeting with families about developmental problems; some set aside a Saturday morning, others an evening. But conferences should be scheduled in a time of quiet when the physician can give the parents full attention. Such conferences should be conducted in an office where the door can be closed for privacy. There is nothing more insulting to parents than to meet with a physician in a bustling waiting room, and there be told that their child is retarded, has cerebral palsy, or has a similar problem.

STAFFING A PARENT CONFERENCE

The question of which professionals should be included in a parent conference should be based on some rationale. It is most logical to include professionals who know the data that will be imparted to the family. Ideally, these should be persons who have a rapport with the family, so that the situation will be more comfortable for the parents and it will be easier for them to hear what is being said. The professionals who attend should also be people who can deal with the emotions which are likely to arise at a parent conference. The professional who is included may be from any discipline, such as speech pathology, physical therapy, psychology, social work, or nursing.

The child's primary physician is almost always required to conduct the parent conference. The question really becomes whether the physician should conduct the parent conference alone, or whether other professionals should be involved. Although there may be some exceptions, it is usually the physician who is most completely informed about the medical issues which relate to the child. Even if medical issues are not the primary areas of discussion, medical questions almost inevitably arise. Also, if the physician has been involved with the family for any length of time, he or she should have the kind of relationship with the family which will make the conference more comfortable for them.

The major question facing each physician is whether he or she feels able to deal with the emotions that are likely to result from a parent conference. Will the physician be able to deal with the parents' sadness, anger, and guilt? If so, he or she may well be able to conduct the parent conference alone. If not, someone else should probably sit in to help deal with the parents' affective responses.

THE SECOND PARENT CONFERENCE

There should always be more than one conference with each family, although the most important is probably the first.

As a rule, a second conference should generally be scheduled within a week or two following the first; usually, about 30 minutes is adequate time for this follow-up conference. As has been noted, the parents may have been so overwhelmed during the first conference that they did not hear much of what was said; they also may not have understood some of the information, or they may have distorted it.

One of the important goals of the second parent conference is for the physician to find out from the family their understanding of what was previously discussed. One comfortable way of eliciting that information is to ask the parents how they are telling grandparents, neighbors or friends about their child's condition. This avoids giving parents the feeling that they are being tested or examined. It also raises the very real issue of the reaction of other people they care about—their family, friends, neighbors, and colleagues. Physicians should be aware that sometimes families may need more than one follow-up conference.

ONGOING CONFERENCES

A third category of conferences can be called ongoing conferences. It is important that the physician meet periodically with the parents without the child being present, and at a time when there is no acute medical stress. Ongoing conferences give parents a chance to discuss how their child is proceeding. When an infant or very young child has been diagnosed as developmentally disabled, meeting with the parents every three to four months for a 15-minute session is usually adequate; perhaps meeting every six to 12 months will be sufficient, depending on how the family and child are adjusting.

The goals of the ongoing conferences are slightly different from the initial and secondary parent conferences. This is because, with time, concerns will arise which were not present initially. These might involve questions about education or preschool classroom settings for the child.

The parents will eventually have questions about how the child is responding to therapy or to prescribed medications. Questions may arise about whether the child should continue to live at home. The ongoing conferences give the physician the opportunity to monitor how the family is being affected by the handicapped child. The physician can learn during the ongoing conferences the status of the marital situation, and whether the entire family is functioning adequately. If the family is functioning suboptimally, the physician may want to intervene.

These ongoing conferences also help let the family know that the physician will stand with them and help them deal with their child's problem. Even though the condition is not curable and won't go away, even though the physician may not know the precise cause of the problem, involvement in ongoing conferences tells the parents that they will have help and support over the course of time.

TERMINATING PARENT CONFERENCES

Eventually the question arises as to when conferences should be terminated.

One criterion is whether the physician has or has not given the parents all the information they should have. The physician also needs to have answered all the significant questions of the family before conferences are terminated. And finally, parent conferences should not be ended when the family is still in some sort of emotional shock. The parents should have the opportunity to pull themselves together before they must face the world on their own. Physicians have to be somewhat sensitive as to how much any one person or any couple can assimilate, deal with, and understand in one sitting. The parents' affective responses in terms of how much they are hearing and understanding, or how overwhelmed they seem to be, will be landmarks for the physician in deciding when to terminate.

SUMMARY

The parent conference is a time for the physician: to impart information; to help the family deal with their emotions; and to aid the family in dealing with the affect of diagnosis, and of the child on the family. It is also a time to help set the stage for a long-term relationship between parents and physician, for the physician will give the family with a handicapped child far more service than the family of a normal, healthy child.

While there are some written materials which may be helpful to parents (see the Bibliography for this chapter), the presence of the physician is the most critical factor for a family. A busy physician might well ask, "Why conduct a parent conference? Why not just write out information about the child, hand it to the family on a sheet of paper, and let them read it at home?"

The physician should instead think about what a difference he or she can make through his or her physical presence. This should help clarify the important aspects of what a physician can and should do during parent conferences with families who have developmentally disabled children.

APPENDIX A

Parent Conference Checklist

(For use with the videotaped parent conference demonstration)

Six Goals of the First Parent Conference

_____ Informing parents of diagnosis and etiology
_____ Eliciting parents' cognitive and emotional responses
_____ Responding to parents' questions and concerns
_____ Assessing affect on the family
_____ Clarifying the physician's future role
_____ Imparting a realistic perspective

Parental Reactions	and	*Physician's Appropriate Response*
_____	Parents appear overwhelmed	_____
_____	Parents mis-hear physician	_____
_____	Parents show denial	_____
_____	Parents appear sad	_____
_____	Parents direct anger inappropriately	_____
_____	Parents demonstrate guilt	_____

BIBLIOGRAPHY

Carek, D. J. Focus on affect: The pediatrician and empathic confrontation. *Clinical Pediatrics,* 1978, *17,* 574–578.

Gayton, W. F. Management problems of mentally retarded children and their families. *Pediatric Clincs of North America,* 1975, *22,* 561–570.

Grant, W. W. What parents of a chronically ill or dysfunctioning child always want to know but may be afraid to ask. *Clinical Pediatrics,* 1978, *17,* 915–917.

Hersey, W. J., and Lapidus, K. R. Restoring the balance. *Pediatric Clinics of North America,* 1973, *20,* 221–231.

Martin, H. P. Developmental problems of childhood. In C. H. Kempe, H. K. Silver, and D. O'Brien (Eds.). *Current pediatric diagnosis and treatment* (5th ed.). Los Altos, Calif.: Lange, 1978, 624–635.

Pearson, P. H. The physician's role in diagnosis and management of the mentally retarded. *Pediatric Clinics of North America,* 1968, *15,* 835–859.

Zuckerberg, H. D., and Snow, G. R. What do parents expect from the physician: A resume of recent opinions. *Pediatric Clinics of North America,* 1968, *15,* 861–870.

SUGGESTED READINGS FOR PARENTS

Several pamphlets and books for parents of developmentally delayed children are listed below. As a part of parent counseling, the physician may wish to recommend some of these publications to parents seeking more information about their child's problems and special needs.

Barnard, K. E., and Erickson, M. *Teaching children with developmental problems: A family care approach.* St. Louis: C. V. Mosby, 1976.

Finnie, N. *Handling the young cerebral palsied child at home.* New York: E. P. Dutton, 1975.

Gordon, I. *Baby learning through baby play: A parent's guide for the first two years.* New York: St. Martin's Press, 1970.

Hasitavej, R. *How to live with and overcome the problems of mental retardation: Questions and answers for parents and counselors.* New York: Exposition, 1975.

Hoffman, S. *Infant stimulation: A pamphlet for parents of multiply-handicapped children.* Denver: Colorado Department of Education, 1973.

Krajicek, M. J., Turner, C., Barnes, P., and Borthick, W. A. *Stimulation activities guide for children from birth to five years.* Denver: JFK Child Development Center, 1973.

Levy, J. *The baby exercise book* (Rev. ed.). New York: Random House, 1975.

Love, H. *The mentally retarded child and his family.* Springfield, Ill.: Thomas, 1973.

Mather, J. *Make the most of your baby: A booklet for parents of mentally retarded infants and preschool children.* Dallas: National Association for Retarded Citizens, 1974.

Smith, D. W., and Wilson, A. A. *The child with Down's syndrome (mongolism): For parents, physicians, and persons concerned with his education and care.* Philadelphia: W. B. Saunders Company, 1973.

PART III

Chapter 15

Goal
To make physicians aware of their role in the educational assessment of the child with developmental disabilities and/or mental retardation.

Objectives
At the end of this chapter, the physician should be able to:
- describe the significance of Public Law 94-142 for children with developmental disabilities and/or mental retardation;
- describe the relevance of physicians and educators working together in the identification and evaluation of children needing an individual education program;
- explain the physician's role in relation to the educational assessment process.

COMPREHENSIVE APPROACH TO FOLLOW-UP

EDUCATIONAL PLANNING

PART I: AN OVERVIEW

By
JOHN MELCHER

I. Importance of Early Assessment
   A. The first six years of life are the years of greatest growth and development.
   B. Public Law 94-142 and various state laws mandate free public education for all handicapped children.
II. Need for an Integrated Approach
   A. Physicians and educators must develop an integrated approach to service delivery.
   B. Cooperation is necessary through the steps of identification, diagnosis, assessment of abilities, and development of an educational program.
III. Identification
   A. Physicians are primary referral sources.
   B. Parents, siblings, day care workers, neighbors, and friends are other valuable referral sources.
   C. Such community programs as Child Find and Kindergarten Round-Ups also locate handicapped children.
IV. Diagnosis
   A. Treatment must never be based solely on screening or identification information.
   B. A complete diagnostic profile includes information on the child's:
      1. Cognitive and reasoning skills;
      2. Gross motor skills;
      3. Fine motor skills;
      4. Receptive and expressive language abilities;
      5. Personal and self-help skills;
      6. Social interaction skills.
V. Educational Assessment
   A. Design of an educational program requires complete information about the child's strengths, weaknesses, and needs.
   B. Formal evaluations by physicians and other health care professionals are combined with informal evaluations by parents and teachers to provide a profile of the child's abilities.
VI. Development of an Individual Educational Program (IEP)
   A. An IEP is required for each handicapped child by federal law.
   B. The IEP must include the following:
      1. A statement of the child's performance level;
      2. Educational goals for the year;
      3. Short-term objectives for each goal;
      4. A time-line for each objective;
      5. A plan for evaluating progress toward each objective;
      6. A provision for updating and revising the IEP.

VII. Overview of the Roles of the Physician
    A. One major role of the physician is as a medical diagnostician.
    B. A second role is that of a referral source.
    C. The physician may also serve as a consultant resource.
    D. The physician is an authority figure and can be a child advocate.
VIII. Summary

IMPORTANCE OF EARLY ASSESSMENT

People everywhere are becoming more aware of the very special needs of developmentally handicapped children. No longer is it just the physician or the teacher of a special education class who is conscious of the extreme importance of early identification and treatment of the handicapped. The first six years of a child's life are now known to be the years of greatest growth and development; if a handicap can be identified and treated during these critical years, the outcome is most often better than it would be if intervention were delayed. Indeed, appropriate early intervention can even prevent secondary problems or complications from developing.

Today, handicapped children, who at one time would have been considered "lucky" to be offered any form of education, have a legislatively-mandated right to receive needed services. A federal law, Public Law 94-142, guarantees free public education for all handicapped children and requires that each child be placed in an educational program appropriate to his or her needs. In addition, 35 states have passed similar legislation.

NEED FOR AN INTEGRATED APPROACH

Society's heightened awareness of the educational needs of handicapped children, as evidenced by legislation and the services for which it provides, has fostered a new relationship between health care professionals and the education community. In order to provide handicapped children with the best possible chance of correcting or overcoming their disabilities, physicians and educators must work together and offer an integrated approach to service delivery. There must be cooperation throughout the process, including the steps of identification of children, diagnosis, assessment of needs and abilities, and development of an appropriate educational program.

IDENTIFICATION

An important first step, one requiring the integration of medical and educational services, involves the identification of children needing those services. Physicians, of course, are a primary referral source, since their diagnostic procedures often identify conditions that mean the child needs special educational services. Well child check-ups and periodic screening are especially vital for infants and preschool-age children who are not routinely seen by school teachers or others who might note a potential handicap.

Parents and siblings are also important referral sources, and a parent's concern that "something is wrong" should never be ignored. Similarly, day care workers, neighbors, or friends of the parents are sometimes responsible for pointing out a possible abnormality.

Mass screening programs represent a community's systematic effort to identify children in need of special attention. Child Find programs, Kindergarten Round-Ups, and routine screening in public health clinics are all important identification modes. These activities often involve the cooperation of professionals from many different fields and provide information that is essential to the development of a successful intervention approach.

DIAGNOSIS

When a child has been identified as having a potential problem, further evaluation and diagnosis are necessary. Remediation efforts or treatment must *never* be based solely on information compiled during the screening or identification stage.

Formal diagnostic evaluations should be performed by physicians, audiologists, psychologists, social workers, and others as deemed necessary for the individual child. Equally valuable evaluations are given by the parents, teachers, peers, and others who have information regarding the child's daily performance and special problems. A complete diagnostic profile, therefore, includes information on the child's functioning and any abnormalities in the following areas:

1. cognitive and reasoning skills;
2. gross motor skills;
3. fine motor skills;
4. receptive and expressive language abilities;
5. personal and self-help skills;
6. social interaction skills, involving both adults and peers.

EDUCATIONAL ASSESSMENT

After diagnostic procedures have confirmed and identified the handicapping condition, further assessment is necessary so that a program of therapy or special training can be designed to meet the child's educational needs. Stating that the child has congenital hearing loss or gross motor impairment is meaningless in an educational setting unless information is also provided on the extent of the handicaps and on the child's specific strengths, weaknesses, and needs.

Educational assessment includes both formal and informal evaluations. Physicians and other health care professionals who performed the diagnostic procedures are asked to supply data about the child's condition, potential for improvement, and required therapies. This information on the child's abilities and deficits is then combined with informal evaluations provided by the parents, teachers, and others to provide an accurate and complete profile of the child's status in each of the six areas listed above.

DEVELOPMENT OF AN INDIVIDUAL EDUCATIONAL PROGRAM

After all the assessment data have been collected and specific areas of educational need identified, the child's case manager develops an Individual Education Program (IEP) for that child. The IEP, a requirement of the previously-mentioned Public Law 94-142, must include:

1. a statement of the child's current level of educational performance;
2. educational goals for the year;
3. specific short-term instructional objectives which will assist the child in meeting each goal;
4. a time-line which specifies when activities will commence, how long they will last, and the approximate date each objective will be met;
5. a plan for evaluating performance and determining when each objective is met;
6. a provision for updating and revising the IEP.

Thus, the IEP represents a strategy for utilizing resources to help a child develop certain competencies and master certain skills. The significance of this plan is that it is tailor-made for each child and is based on that child's individual abilities and needs. It should also be noted that the IEP must take into consideration the role of the parent in the teaching process. Effective parental involvement is to be encouraged, since the parents are, in fact, the major teachers, and their participation will determine the success or failure of the program.

OVERVIEW OF THE ROLES OF THE PHYSICIAN

The primary care physician plays a number of very important roles in educational assessment. He or she may not be the one to write the instructional objectives or oversee their implementation, but the physician provides necessary information and functions on many levels throughout the educational program.

One role of the physician is as a medical diagnostician, for physicians (and other health care professionals) must perform diagnostic evaluations and provide the data necessary for determining what services a child needs. These hard data are necessary so that adequate programs can be developed. Participation on this level should be provided on a continuing basis.

The physician frequently also serves as a referral source; the physician is often the one who first identifies a problem and refers the child for further assessment and educational intervention. The importance of referrals to appropriate professionals or agencies cannot be overemphasized, and the physician must not assume sole responsibility for the child's treatment. Indeed, the physician would do a great disservice to the child and his or her family to try to be a "soloist," since the handicapped child is eligible for a variety of services mandated by federal and state law.

A third role of the physician is as a consultant resource. The physician must be available to provide ongoing consultation services to school personnel. He or she must actively participate, whenever necessary, in the development of the child's educational plan so that the IEP is appropriate and meets the child's needs. Likewise, the physician must reevaluate the child periodically in order to check for medical progress after the IEP is implemented.

And finally, physicians have the role of authority figure and child advocate. Physicians are generally perceived as figures of authority by parents, school personnel, and members of the community in general. Thus, the physician must serve to educate the parents on the nature of their child's disability, on the special services which are available, and on their child's legal rights to educational programs. Similarly, the physician must function as an advocate for the child in the development of public policy and support for the handicapped.

SUMMARY

Effective intervention and treatment of handicapped children require active cooperation of education and health care personnel. This relationship can be a successful one if all involved agree:

1. to have professional respect for others working on the case;
2. to share relevant data with those who need it for planning and program implementation;
3. to divide responsibilities and accept the ability of others to perform their tasks;
4. to work to integrate services so that the focus is on the child's welfare and on what can be done to assist both the child and his or her family.

PART II: THE PHYSICIAN'S ROLE

By
PETER S. FANNING, Ed.D.

I. Introduction
   The physician can define for the schools a child's medical condition, can explain whether that condition is static or progressive, can state what can be done for the child medically, and can outline implications for learning.
II. Conveying Medical Information
   A. Because professionals from other disciplines may not understand technical medical language, the physician may wish to describe the child's condition instead of providing a diagnostic label.
   B. Medical findings should always be related to their implications on school activities.
III. Methods of Communication
   A. Before giving information to schools, the physicians should ensure that the child's parents understand the information to be conveyed and have no objections.
   B. Because of open records laws, findings should be stated in supportable and objective terms.
   C. A simple report can be conveyed in a letter.
   D. Complex findings may require a meeting between the physician and school personnel.
IV. Requesting Teacher Feedback
   A. The teacher can be asked for feedback regarding the child's progress.
   B. The teacher can be told that the physician is available for telephone questions or consultations.
V. Summary

INTRODUCTION

Part One of this chapter has included a description of PL 94-142, which requires educational opportunities for every handicapped child. One premise of the lesson has been that the physician's involvement is necessary if that education is to be optimized. This portion of the chapter will address more specifically the role of the primary care physician in the educational process. The physician can define for the school the medical condition a child has, can explain whether that condition is static or progressive, can state what can be done medically to correct that condition (or conversely, what cannot be done), and can outline what implications of the condition there are for the child's learning.

CONVEYING MEDICAL INFORMATION

The first role mentioned involves conveying medical information. For example, consider the case of a child with a hearing loss. The physician can tell the school the medical condition a child has, tion, surgery, and/or amplification. If a child has congenital cataracts and there is macular damage, the physician can tell the school that nothing can be done medically to correct the condition. When dealing with a child who has seizures or who is hyperactive, the physician can inform the school that there are medications which can be helpful. In other words, the physician can pass along medical knowledge so that the school can plan the most appropriate education for the child.

A word of caution should be interjected at this point. Misunderstandings can arise when professionals from other disciplines may not understand the technical and medical language that the physician might use. For example, the term "epilepsy" may frighten some teachers who may have misconceptions about the condition. Another teacher might be anxious about a child who is diagnosed as having a psychiatric problem. Therefore, it might be best in some cases to *describe* the child's condition instead of providing a diagnostic label. At any rate, when communicating with school personnel, the physician should use caution and attempt to put information into readily-understandable language. In addition, medical findings should always be related to their implications upon school activities.

METHODS OF COMMUNICATION

Next this chapter will consider how the physician can best communicate information about a child to the schools. First, however, it should be noted that confidentiality must always be one of the physician's considerations. Before giving the school *any* information about a child, the physician should always make sure the parents understand the information to be conveyed and have no objections. Second, the physician should be aware of open records laws which give parents access to written information. Therefore, anything the physician writes should be stated in supportable and objective terms rather than subjective or judgmental terms.

If the physician's report is simple or if it is negative in the sense that there is little which can be done for a child medically, it is probably sufficient for the physician to simply send a letter to the school.

If the physician's medical information is complex or has implications for the teaching-learning process, it will probably be best for the physician to discuss the case with the school. Because physicians do not have time to attend all staffings and IEP team meetings regarding a child,

alternate communication approaches will have to be made in many cases.

One option which might be considered is a telephone call to the school. That call should probably be either to the principal, to the school nurse, or to the director of special education for the school district. This call will generally be most effective if the physician talks with one of these team members. If one of these individuals feels that the physician should talk directly with the child's teacher, they will arrange such contact.

Ideally, of course, the physician can meet in person with school personnel; certainly if a case is complex, the physician will want to request such a meeting. This sort of meeting can be scheduled, perhaps, over breakfast or at some other time suitable both to the physician and to school personnel, who also have a full schedule.

REQUESTING TEACHER FEEDBACK

The physician may wish to ask the child's teacher for feedback on the child's progress. The teacher can be told that the physician will put his or her information together with the feedback received from the child's parents; then on the basis of the physician's observations, a decision will be made as to whether or not medication or treatment should be changed. In addition to asking the teacher's help in this manner, the physician will probably want to let the teacher know he or she is available for telephone questions or consultations.

SUMMARY

In summary, this chapter has urged physicians to become involved in educational planning for handicapped children. In this way the physician can make a real difference in the educational progress of these children.

BIBLIOGRAPHY

Battle, C. U. The role of the pediatrician as ombudsman in the health care of the young handicapped child. *Pediatrics*, 1972, *50*, 916–922.

Guralnick, M. J. (Ed.). *Early intervention and the integration of handicapped and non-handicapped children.* Baltimore: University Park Press, 1977.

Jacobs, F., and Walker, D. Pediatricians and the Education for All Handicapped Children Act of 1975 (Public Law 94-142). *Pediatrics,* 1978, *61,* 135–137.

Jordan, J. B., and Dailey, R. F. (Eds.). *Not all little wagons are red.* Reston, Va.: Council for Exceptional Children, 1973.

McDaniels, G. Successful programs for young handicapped children. *Educational Horizons,* 1977, *56,* 26–27.

Minnesota Department of Education. *Early childhood education in six midwest states: Program administration and policy development.* St. Paul: Author, 1977. (Bulletin No. 9263)

Wynne, S., Ulfelder, L. S., and Dakof, G. *Mainstreaming and early childhood education: Review and implications of research.* Washington, D.C.: Office of Education, 1975.

Chapter 16

Goal   To make physicians aware of the general types of community services available for families with handicapped children, and to encourage physicians to become appropriately involved with locating these services.

Objectives   At the end of this chapter, the physician should be able to:
- discuss the general types of community services available for families with handicapped children;
- explain how helping to locate these services can actually save the physician time in the long run;
- state short-cuts to locate community resources.

COMMUNITY RESOURCES

By
DONALD E. COOK, M.D.

I. Introduction
  A. Families with a handicapped child may need special assistance from the primary care physician and the community.
  B. Appendix A has been prepared by the mother of a child with Down Syndrome to help convey an understanding of what community resources can mean to families with handicapped children.
II. General Assistance Categories
  A. Appendix B divides community resources into eight general categories: counseling and self-help, knowledge of resources, financial assistance for health care, income maintenance, housing, education, day care, and recreation.
  B. The tutor has been requested to provide telephone numbers for the agencies listed in Appendix B.
III. The Physician's Role
  While many families can locate needed services without the assistance of the primary care physician, the low-functioning family may need help in obtaining services.
IV. Eliciting Family Need
  A. A common misconception is that families who need help will ask for it; the physician should be alert for nuances from families with a handicapped child.
  B. Even if families have stated that they do not need assistance, the physician should check at periodic intervals to see if the family's needs have changed.
  C. Questions regarding family needs should be phrased tactfully.
V. Summary

INTRODUCTION

Raising a handicapped child can be not only stressful, but may cause severe financial hardships. Therefore, families with a handicapped child may require extra assistance from both the physician and the community. The purpose of this chapter is to make the primary care physician aware of the kinds of community services which are available for families. To provide an understanding of what community services can mean to families with handicapped children, Appendix A has been prepared by the mother of a child with Down Syndrome.

GENERAL ASSISTANCE CATEGORIES

Appendix B has been provided to illustrate the general kinds of assistance programs available in most locales. It divides areas of help for families into eight categories: counseling and self-help, knowledge of resources, financial assis-

221

tance for health care, income maintenance, housing, education, day care, and recreation. The course tutor has been asked to provide telephone numbers for the local agencies and groups listed.

THE PHYSICIAN'S ROLE

Many physicians believe that they cannot spare the time in a busy practice to become involved with locating community resources, and that finding these services should be left to the individual families involved. Of course, many families are capable of seeking help from the appropriate agencies and following through what can be a maze of requirements.

However, other families may be unable to find help. This would be especially true of the low-functioning family, where the parents might not have the initiative to seek help. The physician who sees a family with problems which might prevent the parents from finding help should probably become involved; this involvement may significantly improve the level of family functioning.

ELICITING FAMILY NEED

One common misconception among physicians and other professionals is that families who need help will ask for it. This is not necessarily true. Some families, of course, will ask for assistance, but others will not—for a variety of reasons. Some families consider asking for help a sign of weakness; they may be too proud to admit that they need financial help, for example. Therefore, the physician should be alert for nuances and hints

from families with handicapped children. If the physician is unsure whether a family needs help, the parents probably should be asked directly. Even if a family has stated on previous occasions that they do not need aid, the physician might check at periodic intervals to see if their needs have changed.

Because blunt, direct questions from the physician such as, "Do you have financial problems? Do you need financial aid?" may draw a negative response even when the family could use help, the physician might consider how such questions can be tactfully phrased.

SUMMARY

The purpose of this chapter has been to acquaint the primary care physician with the kinds of community resources available for the families of handicapped children, and to encourage the physician to become involved with finding these services when necessary. Two final points should be considered. First, the physician who is unfamiliar with community services can take a short-cut by establishing contact with someone who knows these services well—like a public health nurse, a psychologist, a social worker, or a citizen-advocate.

Finally, if the physician helps families obtain needed services, it will save that physician time in the long run. An unresolved problem can lead to parents calling the physician again and again for help with problems which could be handled more appropriately by a community agency. In addition, unresolved problems can slow the development of a handicapped child, leading to the need for more intervention from the primary care physician.

APPENDIX A*

It's traumatic to learn you have given birth to a handicapped child. I know, because my son was born 14 years ago with Down Syndrome. Parents in such a situation feel a combination of fear, guilt, and loneliness; other common feelings include a desire to escape, helplessness, and general depression. Most parents eventually work through these feelings, although unfortunately a few do not.

In my experience, the greatest support for families just discovering they have a handicapped or retarded child comes from another family or individual who has had the same experience. During the initial adjustment period, it helps to see that another family in the same situation has not crumbled or been shamed into seclusion. It is helpful to learn that their handicapped child has grown, learned, and become a very important part of the family. It helps to know that siblings have accepted the handicapped child, and have learned a kind of empathy and understanding that few young people acquire today. Through contact with those who have "been there," parents can learn that what was devastating at first has helped another family find a special niche in life, and has made them feel responsible to help the world understand not only their handicapped child, but other handicapped children as well.

Even after the period of initial adjustment, contact with other parents can still be extremely helpful to the family with a handicapped child. Advocacy groups can help a family locate and adjust to various programs, and can help siblings accept and understand their handicapped brother or sister. In addition, parents can band together to establish needed programs.

Today the emphasis is on keeping the handicapped child in the home; to achieve this, families must receive community services assistance. These services frequently start with the primary care physician, because the physician is the first professional involved with a new life.

It is comforting to a family to find that their physician not only cares, but is interested enough in the child and family to inform him- or herself about community resources. Even if the physician's knowledge of these resources is limited, the personal involvement means a lot to the family.

The day is past when the physician can say to the parents of a retarded boy, for example: "Just take him home and love him," or "Put him in an institution." Now the physician can say that infant stimulation programs and parent support groups are available, and that the sooner these are begun, the better. If needed programs are not available, parents can be encouraged to join with others in advocacy groups to help make them a reality.

The physician can be the first to tell parents that federal law mandates—and most states have laws that require—an appropriate education for handicapped children. The parents can be told that their child is guaranteed the same educational opportunities available to all children.

The physician can let the parents know that the future for the handicapped looks brighter. Each year more employment opportunities are opening up, and there are increasing numbers of community residential centers for the time when a child can no longer live at home.

Handicapped people and their families have the right to the same opportunities and services as all citizens. Parents and physicians together have the obligation to ensure that these services are not only available, but that they are utilized appropriately. Our mutual decisions through the early days and years in the lives of handicapped or retarded children determine whether they will become part of the community—or castoffs.

---

*Adapted from remarks by Alice Kitt, former president of the Colorado Association for Retarded Citizens.

APPENDIX B

General Assistance Categories

Categories of Help Provided	Nonprofit and Advocacy Groups	Governmental Programs
1. Counseling and Self-Help		
	a. Association for Retarded Citizens Phone:_____	a. Mental Health Centers, State Department of Mental Health Phone:_____
	b. Association for Children with Learning Disabilities Phone:_____	b. State Department of Social Services Phone:_____
	c. United Cerebral Palsy Association Phone:_____	c. Handicapped or Crippled Children's Program, State Department of Health Phone:_____
	d. Society for Autistic Children Phone:_____	d. Public Health (Visiting) Nurse, State Department of Health Phone:_____
	e. Epilepsy Association Phone:_____	
	f. Spina Bifida Parents' Association Phone:_____	
	g. Centers for the Deaf and Blind Phone:_____	
2. Knowledge of Resources		
	a. United Way Phone:_____	a. State Developmental Disabilities Council Phone:_____
	b. All the groups listed under Number 1	b. State Department of Social Services Phone:_____
		c. State Department of Health Phone:_____
		d. Area Health Education Center Phone:_____

Categories of Help Provided	Nonprofit and Advocacy Groups	Governmental Programs
3. Financial Assistance for Health Care		
	a. March of Dimes/ Birth Defects Phone:_____	a. Medical Assistance (Medicaid), State Department of Social Services Phone:_____
	b. Shriners Hospitals for the Handicapped Phone:_____	b. Handicapped or Crippled Children's Program, State Department of Health Phone:_____
		c. Public Health (Visiting) Nurse, State Department of Health Phone:_____
		d. County Department of Social Services Phone:_____
4. Income Maintenance		
		a. Supplemental Security Income, District Social Security Office Phone:_____
5. Housing		
		a. State Department of Institutions (or Department of Social Services or Housing) Phone:_____
		b. Local Housing Authority Phone:_____
		c. Foster Homes, State Department of Social Services Phone:_____

Categories of Help Provided	Nonprofit and Advocacy Groups	Governmental Programs
6. Education		a. Division of Special Education, State Department of Education Phone:_____
		b. Pupil Service Department, Local School District Phone:_____
		c. Boards of Cooperative Educational Services Phone:_____
		d. Area Health Education Centers Phone:_____
7. Day Care	a. State Day Care Association Phone:_____	a. State and Local Departments of Social Services Phone:_____
		b. County Departments of Social Services Phone:_____
8. Recreation	a. YMCA Phone:_____	a. Local Departments of Parks and Recreation Phone:_____
	b. YWCA Phone:_____	
	c. American Red Cross Phone:_____	
	d. Boy Scouts of America Phone:_____	
	e. Girl Scouts of America Phone:_____	
	f. Association for Retarded Citizens Phone:_____	

PART IV

Chapter 17 ⸻⸻⸻⸻⸻⸻⸻⸻⸻⸻⸻⸻⸻⸻⸻⸻

Goal   To review the evaluation and referral procedures recommended in this
training program, and to introduce students to the practicum period.

Objectives   At the end of this chapter, the physician should be able to:
   • state the evaluation and referral procedures recommended for a child
     who is suspected of developmental delays;
   • discuss the interim practices which it is requested that students com-
     plete;
   • state the purposes and procedures of the practicum meeting.

PRACTICUM

By
WILLIAM K. FRANKENBURG, M.D.

I. A Diagnostic Review
This final lesson will include an in-class, step-by-step review of diagnostic evaluation and referral procedures led by the tutor.

II. The Practicum Period
A. During the practicum period, students are requested to practice the procedures learned in this training program, and to evaluate six or more cases before meeting again with the tutor.
B. If problems are encountered, students are urged to contact the tutor.

III. The Practicum Meeting
A. At the practicum meeting, the tutor will evaluate students' proficiencies in performing tests and procedures, and will give students the opportunity to discuss cases in their practices.
B. Persons successfully completing the course will receive certificates of competence.

IV. Summary

A DIAGNOSTIC REVIEW

This is the final chapter in the training program; it will consist of an in-class review of what students have learned regarding pediatric developmental diagnosis.

The tutors for the videotaped program have been asked to take students enrolled through the case of a child who was suspect on developmental screening. Students will be asked to decide, step by step, what action they would take regarding conducting evaluations or referring to other professionals. The results of those evaluations or referrals will be presented to students by the tutor—also step by step.

THE PRACTICUM PERIOD

This educational program and the example case presented in class by the tutor have demonstrated how the physician might evaluate children who are developmentally suspect. As in the learning of any new procedure, the students now need to apply the aforementioned to cases in their practices before a high degree of skill will be acquired. It is for this reason that this first part of the training program is completed with the request that the students practice the various procedures that were taught, and that they evaluate six cases or more before meeting again with the tutor. If problems are encountered during this interim period, students are encouraged to contact the tutor to request assistance.

THE PRACTICUM MEETING

The final portion of the training program is a practicum meeting, to be scheduled with the tutor. At this final session, the tutor will evaluate students' proficiencies in performing various tests and procedures, and will give students an opportunity to discuss cases that they have evaluated in their practices. Persons successfully completing the initial classroom instruction, the practicum, and the follow-up practicum session will receive certificates of competence.

SUMMARY

Parents, professionals, and the lay public—all of whom have long been dismayed at the lack of physician training in developmental diagnosis—will be seeking the assistance of physicians who complete this training program on behalf of children with developmental problems. This brief course has been designed to teach participants the essentials of the diagnostic procedure. As in much of medicine, no one expects the primary care physician to know all of the answers; but if the physician encounters a problem that he or she cannot solve, it is hoped that appropriate help will be sought so that the child can be helped to reach his or her fullest capacity.

Chapter 18

In concluding this text, it is appropriate to review the major goals of this program. It is hoped that this text, used in combination with the videotaped lessons, practice sessions, and classroom discussions, will enable the physician to become more adept at identifying, evaluating, and referring developmentally delayed children. The physician must assume the primary responsibility for detecting delays and for ensuring that needed diagnostic, therapeutic, and follow-up services are provided.

Certain screening tests should be performed on all children seen by a primary care physician. Once delayed or suspect children are identified, the physician should perform a diagnostic evaluation, which includes compiling a profile of the child's medical history, examining the child physically, and either conducting extensive medical assessments or referring the child to specialists for such tests. Results of laboratory tests and reports from consultants are then reviewed and integrated into a comprehensive diagnosis and treatment plan.

The physician who serves as case manager will also oversee and coordinate follow-up activities including: conducting parent conferences, developing an educational intervention strategy, and possibly assisting the family in locating community resources.

Whether assuming the active role of case manager or simply serving as a medical consultant, a physician concerned about the welfare of young children can profit from a review of this text and the accompanying video presentations. Skillful and accurate evaluation of children, however, comes only with practice; thus this training program must be viewed only as a beginning. It provides guidelines, procedures, and reference materials, but the practicing physician must actually work with children in order to gain skill and confidence in assessing developmental delays, and in planning treatment and needed follow-up services for the handicapped child.

Conclusion

INDEX

Page numbers followed by a "t" refer to tables; numbers followed by an "o" refer to material in chapter openings. *Italics* signify illustrations and reproduced forms.